"A spellbinding account of the author's personal encounter with ovarian cancer. As a registered nurse with 40 years of experience in this field, she manages to convey a strong sense of both the physical and emotional impact of the condition in the context of clinically accurate, helpful information related to its diagnosis and treatment. This book is a must-read for women with gynecologic cancer as well as for those who love and support them."

—Mary Burke, D.N.Sc., R.N.

Views from the Other Side
of the Looking Glass

Views from the Other Side of the Looking Glass

✦

Reflections on My Journey with Ovarian Cancer

Terry Downey

iUniverse, Inc.
New York Lincoln Shanghai

Views from the Other Side of the Looking Glass
Reflections on My Journey with Ovarian Cancer

iUniverse books may be ordered through booksellers or by contacting:

iUniverse
2021 Pine Lake Road, Suite 100
Lincoln, NE 68512
www.iuniverse.com
1-800-Authors (1-800-288-4677)

ISBN-13: 978-0-595-34709-4 (pbk)
ISBN-13: 978-0-595-67144-1 (cloth)
ISBN-13: 978-0-595-79452-2 (ebk)
ISBN-10: 0-595-34709-6 (pbk)
ISBN-10: 0-595-67144-6 (cloth)
ISBN-10: 0-595-79452-1 (ebk)

Printed in the United States of America

Contents

Introduction

It was spring 1944. As I started to stir—half-awake and half-asleep—my eyes seemed to be glued shut. I struggled to open them but they didn't seem to want to obey me. When I could finally open my eyes a little, I could see a glimmer of light entering the room through a gap between the window frame and the window shade. This faint glimmer of light did little to help me to make out my surroundings. I just didn't know where I was. I didn't seem to be where I ought to be—this didn't seem to be the place where I'd gone to sleep the night before. Yet the surroundings were strangely familiar. I'd been here before, but I didn't know where I was now. As I struggled to wake up, nothing seemed to be in the right place! Everything seemed so vague, yet so strangely familiar!

I wondered, "Where am I? How'd I get here? The place had an inexplicable familiarity about it. If I'd been here before, why didn't I know where I was now? As the sun appeared more visibly through the gap between the window frame and the window shade, the surroundings appeared to be more familiar to me. Gradually I began to realize that I was in my bedroom. During the night, as I had often done, I had turned around completely and my head was now at the foot of my bed and I was looking out at the world through partly closed eyes into a reverse image of my bedroom. It was as if I was looking out from the other side of the looking glass. This is how it has been for me since I discovered that I had ovarian cancer and agreed to its treatment.

The day before my journey began was a typical day. I taught nursing students at Bayside College, had lunch with my colleagues, had meetings, and graded tests. After dinner with my family I met with my religious education class in the evening. Then I had the symptom—one that doesn't usually mark the onset of ovarian cancer. I knew that 1 in 59 women would be diagnosed with ovarian cancer and more than half on them who were would die from the disease.

I didn't know it yet but I was about to go someplace where I didn't expect to go. After all I was a nurse. I cared for patients. I didn't expect to become a patient. My life would be turned around completely and I would be looking out from the other side of the looking glass. Gradually the invasion of my body by ovarian cancer would be revealed but I had no reason to suspect its presence yet. As I continued on my journey, I found myself in that strangely familiar place more and more often. My world would never be the same as it was the day before my journey began.

Defining symptoms during the early stages of ovarian cancer are rare. Most women are diagnosed in the late stages. I was more fortunate than most women were. I had a symptom—a symptom that every woman dreads—a defining moment. I will never forget that moment. It changed my life.

Something was wrong—very wrong. Even the receptionist knew it. They would fit me in. Suddenly I was on a high-speed train—going someplace that I didn't want to go. I didn't have a reservation. I didn't have a destination. It didn't matter. I had the symptom. I could come on board.

As the train sped rapidly down the track, my primary care physician arranged an array of appointments with other physicians and various diagnostic tests. Descriptions of the pictures of my inner body didn't verify the presence or absence of cancer. Instead they suggested a diverse assortment of diagnoses. It was like having to choose an answer for a multiple-choice question but choosing the answer that I liked best—most likely a fibroid—wasn't an option.

My surgeon discovered that I was in the first stage of ovarian cancer, not a bad place to be if ovarian cancer is inevitable. My surgeon got it all but the patholo-gist reported that the cell was aggressive. Chemotherapy would be needed after all. After completing a course of chemotherapy with paclitaxel (Taxol) and carbo-platin (Paraplatin), I was invited to take part in a phase III clinical trial. I won the lottery and received cutting edge Radioimmune Therapy.

When I first learned of the likelihood that I had cancer, I thought that my life was over. Then I began to look for information and was dismayed to learn that the ordinary woman couldn't go into a local bookstore and choose from an array of books describing the experience of living with ovarian cancer or any other gynecologic cancer.

I was on the train traveling at breakneck speed to an unknown place and I couldn't find a tour book. As a nurse I had access to books that described an array of cancers, diagnostic tests, and anticancer medications. As an educator I had access to the Internet and could search for information. As a researcher I could evaluate the trustworthiness of the research reports. Although I knew what would happen, I needed my surgeon to tell me, "Yes, this is what will take place." Nothing prepared me for what it would be like if I actually had cancer.

In many ways my journey was less tumultuous than most women's journeys were. My cancer was detected early. My good health enabled me to withstand surgery, chemotherapy and radioimmune therapy readily.

Colleagues who had survived ovarian cancer or other women's cancers heard of my diagnosis and shared their experiences with me. An associate kept me updated on the status of her sister-in-law who had been diagnosed in a later stage of ovarian cancer. She was too sick to undertake the telling of her story. She died. Her husband wants to know, "Why didn't they do the tests? Why didn't they discover this earlier?"

Hearing that early symptoms of ovarian cancer are vague and that a positive test result doesn't indicate the presence of ovarian cancer and a negative test result doesn't indicate the absence of ovarian cancer wasn't comforting. The search for better answers is ongoing.

One year after surgery and diagnosis, I was invited to be a patient teacher for a first year medical student at a world-renowned medical school in the area. She was enrolled in a course entitled Living with a Life Threatening Illness. The opportunity to share a patient's perspective with a future physician enticed me to meet with her weekly for several months and describe my experience.

She learned how difficult it was for me at times to think of myself as a patient and how I created flow sheets and kept records of various events and symptoms as if I was writing about someone else. She also learned how important it was for me to become aware that I had created my own definition of the situation within the context of my unique life experience. This awareness provided me with a new sense of continuity about my journey. It's my hope that sharing my story with other women who are traveling along similar roads will be helpful to them.

1

Learning the Awful Truth

During the first few days of October 2001 I experienced sensations that I hadn't experienced for several years. I thought, "If I didn't know better, I would think that this was PMS (premenstrual syndrome) again." Realizing that the days of PMS were behind me, I quickly dismissed these unwelcome thoughts from my mind. After all menopause had occurred in the spring of 1994. At least I think that is when I think that it ended—in the spring of 1994. I'd been so grateful that menstrual discomfort was behind me. I wouldn't be joyfully anticipating its return.

Menarche—my first menstrual period—arrived at 2:10 PM on Friday December 12, 1947 in the middle of art class. Fortunately school would be out in twenty minutes and I could be home in two minutes. I wouldn't be embarrassed by having to ask to leave class for such a personal moment. Unlike menarche, I'm not able to define a precise moment that menopause—my last menstrual period—occurred. I had to try to remember what events were taking place in my life around the time of my last menstrual periods. Then there was the false alarm to contend with! Nine months without a period! They resumed for several more months before they stopped entirely.

In the beginning some young women have irregular menstrual periods. Unlike other young women mine occurred every 21–23 days and persisted for 5–6 days each cycle. Unless I stayed active, I was very uncomfortable during my periods. Moreover periods accounted for one fourth of my life between menarche and menopause! Premenstrual syndrome was such an integral part of my life that a quick dismissal of any thoughts of PMS all over again was fitting.

Then, at midnight on October 3rd I had some spotting—about a quarter's worth—not enough to worry about! Yeah, right! I knew the drill! Be seen by a physician. But it can't be anything serious—or is it something?

My thoughts went back to January when I saw a new primary physician for the first time. I had actually suggested that maybe I didn't need a Papanicolaou (Pap) smear because I wasn't sexually active and I had at least three consecutive negative examinations. Although my new primary physician was in the same group as my former physician, my medical records weren't available. They were offsite. She was reluctant to listen to my advice and insisted that I have the examination.

During the examination it felt as if she were tugging at my left broad ligament. All that went through my mind was "When will this be over? Will this exam ever end?" When it did come to an end, my physician didn't voice any concerns about her findings.

She recommended a sigmoidoscopy. I was reluctant to submit to a sigmoidoscopy. I said, "I have to think about it." She handed me a kit for collecting and testing stool specimens for "hidden blood" (not visible to the naked eye).

She suggested a bone density study to rule out osteoporosis—a disease in which decreased bone density increases risk for fractures. She asked, "Are you going to do this?" I responded, "I can do this."

I really didn't want the Pap smear but I gave in. I had worked for a year as a nurse's aid in a major teaching hospital in the Northeast in 1954–1955. Pap smears were just being introduced at this time. The hospital policy was that all women would have a Pap smear before being discharged.

One of my responsibilities was bringing women to the examination room and assisting the residents during this procedure. When they wrote the discharge summaries, the residents usually discovered that the women hadn't had the mandatory Pap smear. Often elderly women would be so fatigued after the examination that their discharge would be delayed until the next day. The frequency of delayed discharges in these elderly women upset me.

Another one of my responsibilities was bringing patients to the examination room for sigmoidoscopy and assisting the residents during the procedure. In the 1950s the physician used a rigid metal instrument. Flexible instruments were decades away. A young woman who was my age described what the experience of having this examination was like for her. It had been exhausting and dehumanizing for her. She had said, "It takes all your dignity away." I couldn't imagine what it was like. I didn't want to know.

As these thoughts are flashing through my mind, I have more spotting—another quarter's worth! This is getting serious. Morning is a long way off. I'll call my physician in the morning to make an appointment.

The next day I woke up and got ready to go to work. My plan was to call my physician from work and make an appointment. As I get ready for work, I have some fleeting pink drainage. I think, "Oh, this is only a cyst; it's probably nothing, but I can't ignore it. I know the drill."

I went to work. I had some scant bleeding. It was old. Several times I tried to call my physician's office but the line was busy. This was driving me crazy. "How can their line be busy?" I thought. This has never happened before.

Finally I got through to the receptionist. I said, "I have vaginal bleeding." She took down the necessary information. Then, she said, "Your physician doesn't have an opening but vaginal bleeding is a priority situation. I'm going to put you through to her 'nurse'. She'll fit you in! She has to do this. This is a priority." I was reassured. The receptionist knows what to do.

The 'nurse' said, "She doesn't have any time in her schedule."

I said, "But, I have vaginal bleeding. This is urgent. I need to be seen."

She reiterated, "She has no openings."

Again I said, "I have vaginal bleeding. I need to be seen."

She said, "Well, she has no time to see you."

I was puzzled. I said, "The receptionist said that this is a priority situation, that you would fit me in."

She restated, "She has no openings."

Her failure to find a solution to this dilemma baffled me. My anxiety level was mounting. I asked, "Don't you have nurse practitioners who see patients with urgent problems?"

The 'nurse' said, "Yeah."

I suggested, "Why don't you see if one of them has an opening?"

She responded, "Diane M can see you at 9:00 AM."

I breathed a sigh of relief and hung up.

I arrived on time the following day. While I was still signing in, Diane opened the door to the reception area and called my name.

She brought me to an examining room. I explained, "I had some bleeding, nothing much, but I know that I should have it looked into." After Diane examined me, she said, "I think that it is just a fibroid but I'm going to order a complete blood count (CBC), a thyroid test and a pelvic ultrasound to be sure. We'll let you know the results as soon as they are available." A few days later I learned that the CBC and thyroid test were normal. The ultrasound wasn't scheduled until October 23rd.

The pelvic ultrasound was scheduled at 1:00 PM. Although I wasn't eager to miss class time, I dismissed my class early so that I could start drinking water—ALL 24 OUNCES—and so I would make my appointment on time. This was the only day that I missed any scheduled class time related to my illness.

As I drove to the hospital, I continued drinking and I worried that I'd be late. I arrived on time and had no trouble finding a parking space. I signed in. The receptionist asked, "Did you drink?"

"Oh, yes!"

She directed me to the waiting area.

A few minutes later, Barry called me. He asked, "Did you drink?" As we walked toward the examining room, he explained the procedure. After we entered the room, he handed me a gown and told me to take off everything below the waist and to put on the gown. He said, "I'll be back in a few minutes."

The dark, drab windowless room was small, barely enough space for the examining table and the ultrasound machine. I looked around for a place to put my clothes, my fanny pack, and my reading materials. Space was definitely at a premium. It wasn't easy to find a place to store my belongings.

Barry kept his promise and returned within minutes. The woman who accompanied him was dressed in street attire rather than hospital scrubs. As Barry carried out the ultrasound procedure, the woman explained features of this ultrasound machine that their current ultrasound machine apparently didn't have. At first I thought that Barry was a student and he was learning the ropes. As they proceeded, I became aware that she was a company representative. She was demonstrating the use of a new machine. During the entire procedure, they talked and chewed gum. The gum chewing was constant and annoying. I wondered, "Do they realized how annoying this is, how unprofessional this behavior is?"

The woman showed him how to enter data. She explained how information such as the dimensions of the uterus could be calculated. This information didn't excite me. Later, this information would serve a purpose, but now it didn't matter. I was waiting for my clean bill of health! It never came.

Barry asked questions and the woman provided additional information. The rhythmic gum chewing continued without interruption. I recalled how I had been able to chew gum in junior high school all morning without being caught by my teachers. At noon I would brazenly open my mouth, remove the gum, and pitch it into the wastebasket in front of the teacher. I would make sure that she saw it. She would know that I got away with it. I wondered, "Maybe they were allowed to chew gum in school. Perhaps this was why they did not learn how to chew gum inconspicuously."

I didn't have a good view of the ultrasound screen. I had no idea what they were looking at most of the time. My mind wandered off. I thought of the days that I had assisted during the amniocenteses and ultrasounds at the children's rehabilitation center.

Watching a cute little unborn move about its mother's womb and avoid the obstetrician's needle was definitely a lot more fun.

All parents wanted to know that their developing infants were normal. Most were also curious to know if the little one was a boy or a girl. Some didn't want to know until it was born. This was how it was when I worked in the labor and birth unit in the early 1970s. Each and every time the sex of the unborn was a mystery.

Now, when I arranged for my students to observe a labor and birth, my students always asked, "Do you know what it is?" Expectant parents eagerly shared whether they chose to know or not know the sex of their unborn infant.

I also recalled how the parents learned about the sex of the unborn at the amniocenteses that I observed. Although the obstetrician was reluctant to reveal the sex of the unborn, the radiologist eagerly shared his discovery.

Then, my mind returned to the present. What did Barry and the woman find so interesting? They seemed to be deeply involved in the technical aspects of the procedure and their coordinated gum chewing. I was given a welcome break so that I could empty my bladder.

When I returned, Barry told me that they needed additional views. They would be taken in another area of the radiology department. He offered to have a female assist me with the additional views. I gathered my belongings and followed Barry to another examining room.

Tara came in shortly thereafter and told me what she would be doing. She instructed me to put a probe in place. I had no idea what I was supposed to do but I guess that it was okay because images were being projected on the screen. I could see some of them and recognized some anatomical structures. Tara continued with the ultrasound. It became apparent that she wasn't seeing what she knew that she needed to capture on screen. Beth joined her and assisted her. As soon as they were sure that they had visualized all that they could, they notified the radiologist. After his initial assessment he asked me if I could drink more water. He was attempting to verify that my ovaries couldn't be visualized. As soon as he was certain that the ovaries couldn't be visualized satisfactorily, he ended the examination. However, I thought that only the left ovary couldn't be seen. I didn't realize that the right ovary also couldn't be seen. I suspected that something was wrong but I hoped for the best.

I knew that I needed surgery but I wasn't sure who would do the surgery. At the local hospital where I initially studied nursing, surgeons usually performed hysterectomies. I wondered if gynecologists did also. I wasn't sure. I went to the Internet to search for physicians affiliated with North Shore Medical Center (NSMC). Initially a clear answer to my question did not emerge. Then the *entry Gynecologic Oncologist* seemed to leap off the page. I doubled-clicked and was introduced to a physician whose credentials were remarkable! Dr. D had graduated from Johns Hopkins Medical School and was *Board Certified in Obstetrics and Gynecology and Gynecologic Oncology.* I need look no further. I felt confident that the completion of her medical preparation was recent enough that her knowledge base would be current and yet not so recent that she would lack sufficient experience. Later I would learn that I couldn't have made a better choice.

My primary care physician called me on October 26th to say, "You have endometrial hyperplasia. There is a mass that could be a fibroid or an ovary or a polyp. You need to have a uterine biopsy and a CT Scan."

Dr. B went on to say, "There's nothing to it (the biopsy). It's an office procedure. Do you have a gynecologist?"

"No," I responded, "I have always had my Pap smears done by my regular physician. There is someone—a physician whom I want to see—LD."

"But, she's a surgeon!"

I said, "Yeah, I know." I thought, "This fibroid has to go."

"You need to see a gynecologist first. Do you have a preference?"

"There is a group in the next town—North Shore Gynecologic Associates."

"I'll have Paula call. Would you prefer a woman?"

"Yes!"

"Okay. Don't worry. It's nothing. They do it in the office."

Within the half-hour Paula called back. "Dr. G can see you on November 1st at 3:45 PM. The CT Scan is booked for November 16th at 9:00 AM. You need to go to radiology the day before to pick up the contrast material. Don't forget it. It's important."

I thought, "This is getting serious. Maybe, it's cancer. Maybe, it's not. The GYN oncologist will know!"

The following Thursday I went to see Dr G. When his assistant did the intake screening, she said, "We received a copy of your Pap smear test results from January. It is normal. We couldn't figure out why you were referred to us. When I called, they didn't want to give me any information."

Astounded, I replied, "My doctor told me that I had to have an endometrial biopsy. According to the ultrasound, I could have endometrial hyperplasia or a polyp. I don't know why they won't give you the reports. The ultrasound was done at NSMC. I can call them and ask for them now."

She said, "Oh, we're part of NSMC. Let me see what I can do." When she returned, she told me that she'd been able to get the report. She led me to an examination room and explained how to get ready for the examination.

Dr. G arrived within a few minutes. He was a pleasant older gentleman who put me at ease. He explained the procedure in detail. I knew that after he inserted the vaginal speculum he would clasp my cervix with an Allis clamp to stabilize the uterus while he inserted the biopsy instrument. It sounded so simple.

He initiated the procedure. It seemed to be going as well as an intrusive vaginal procedure could go. When he inserted the vaginal speculum and opened the blades, I winced. He instructed me, "Breathe in and out slowly." I did and I relaxed. I felt a slight pinch of the Allis clamp as he had explained that I would. When he attempted to insert the biopsy instrument, he met resistance. After another try, he said, "I won't try again. I don't want to risk puncturing your uterus." A stenosis or narrowing of the opening of the uterus prevented the insertion of the instrument.

After I got dressed, he spoke to me. Apparently his assistant was able to obtain more information. Dr. G said, "You have cancer. I am going to refer you to Dr D, a GYN oncologist who consults at the Cancer Center. I have absolute confidence in her and I would follow her recommendations without hesitation. I'm going to order a CA 125. When you see Dr. D, you can tell her that you've had a CA 125 already."

His assistant obtained the blood sample. It was late when I returned to the receptionist. She was unable to reach the Cancer Center. She told me that she would call them the next day. She did. My appointment with Dr D was scheduled for November 13th at 2:30 PM. In the meantime, Dr. B called to tell me that I needed to have another test. She told me to call the Magnetic Resonance Imaging (MRI) Center.

The MRI was scheduled for November 3rd. A friend had this procedure a few years ago. In her words "The MRI is terrible. The noise drives you out of your mind." As the day approaches, I wonder how it will be for me.

> Lately I have not been sleeping very well. The tumor is growing inside me and is pressing on my bladder. Getting up several times during the night has become a way of life.

> A construction company has been working on the separation of the storm drain and sewer system in our neighborhood for several weeks now. Every morning at 6:00 AM the workers begin their day by breaking up the pavement and excavating the area where they will work for the day. I've never been a morning person. Now that I'm not sleeping we'll being awakened early by the loud, rhythmic percussion of the jackhammer day after day is unbearable torture. I think, "After this the MRI will probably be a piece of cake."

On November 3rd I was scheduled for the second of three diagnostic tests. No one told me why I needed all three procedures. Later I would learn that each test detects different components of abnormal tissue.

Unlike other imaging procedures, the MRI is based on the water content of tissue and it enables the visualization of tissue without the interference of bone. In other words, it allows the radiologist to see "through bone." Thus, the MRI might allow the radiologist to see the tissue that was hiding out during the ultrasound.

My reason for having this procedure is more practical. The sooner they rule out cancer, the happier I will be.

I found the MRI Imaging Center easily. The Center was tucked away at the top of a hill just off the highway in a residential neighborhood. The landscaping isolated the building and its parking area from the surrounding neighborhood. The large parking area was almost empty. I imagined that it could be quite busy during the week but today was Saturday.

The receptionist welcomed me and gave me some papers to complete. After I returned the completed papers to the receptionist I was led promptly into the examining area. The technician verified that I didn't have anything magnetic in me or on me. Then she provided me with a locker to store my belongings. I was able to wear my own clothes during the procedure. The technicians explained the procedure to me and guided me onto the examining table. They told me to listen to the recording that would tell me when to take a deep breath and when to hold my breath. They inserted an intravenous access line to allow for the injection of gadolinium a contrast material that is used during MRI of the abdomen to decrease signals from stomach and bowel activity.

After being positioning on the table, the procedure began. The table moved me into the hollow tube and out of the hollow tube during the filming. As instructed, I took deep breaths and held my breath in response to the computerized voice. The Imager went to work. They had warned me that the machine would be noisy. My perception that it would be mild in comparison to the jackhammer that woke me up everyday was borne out. I wonder if I would've agreed if I'd had magnetic resonance imaging of the head. Probably not.

After several cycles of pictures, one of the technicians explained that she would now inject the gadolinium. I continued to be drawn into and out of the hollow tube as I try to coordinate taking deep breaths and holding breaths with the "voice."

Finally the procedure was over. The technicians told me to wait in the reception area. After several minutes, the receptionist called me. She gave me the large radiology envelope that contained my films and said, "Take these to your doctor."

As soon as I got home, I looked at my films. What an experience! I've never been good at reading x-rays but I've recognized the obvious. In 1995 following an injury I noticed the fractured bones in my foot before Dr. Evans pointed to them.

I looked at 16 films each containing 9–15 views each. On the first go-round, I saw no recognizable anatomical structures. The womb is the size and shape of a pear. I didn't see anything that even remotely resembled a pear. I thought that I might be looking at some other part of my body—but what body part could it be? It couldn't be my liver! The pictures didn't resemble anything that I had seen in Gray's anatomy. The films had not portrayed any body parts with which I had been familiar.

After looking at the CT Scan films a few weeks later, I took another look at the MRI films. On the second go-round, some of the surrounding anatomy was recognizable. The femoral heads (the large round upper end of the thighbones that fit into the hipbone), spinal vertebrae (the connected bones that form the back), and the iliac crests (the upper portion of the bones that form the pelvis) were familiar. It was then that I realized that what I didn't recognize earlier was the tumor that was growing in me. It was huge.

Dr. D would know what to do. I would see her in ten days.

The following week I obtained copies of the radiologists' reports of the pelvic ultrasound and the MRI and the ultrasound films. I looked at the reports and the films. I realized from the reports that I could have cancer. I just didn't know where it was yet.

The Cancer Center was next door to the former office of the Visiting Nurses Association. I had driven by there several times. I had no reason to pay much attention to the Cancer Center. Today was different. I was going in.

The reception area was inside the main entrance. I was third in line. The receptionist seemed warm and welcoming. When it was my turn, she asked, "Who are you here to see?" She gave me some papers and directed me to an office on the other side of the waiting room. I was fourth in line.

The other side of the reception area was busy with a flurry of activity. The boutique was being moved to another area. The couches were arranged in a square so that people in the waiting area face one another. A huge aquarium with tropical fish separated the reception area from the waiting area. No one was looking at the aquarium.

Several people were sitting in the waiting area. A thin, lanky, pale, sickly looking man lay on the couch. His wife cuddled his head in her lap and stroked him gently. The woman explained to another visitor, "They released him from the hospital today. His port (catheter through which chemotherapy is administered) is plugged. They told us to bring him here so that they could flush it."

A middle-aged woman and a ten-year old boy came from another area to the waiting area. I did not know why they were here. I wondered if children were treated here.

The line did not seem to move very fast. I ask myself, "What am I doing here? I don't have cancer." I had obtained the Ultrasound and the MRI (Magnetic Resonance Imaging) films and reports. I had looked at the films and I had read the reports. I was carrying the films and reports with me.

I wasn't able to interpret the films but I knew that the pelvic structures were distorted. If it weren't for the clearly delineated rounded heads of the femurs (thighbones) and rounded upper pelvic bones, I wouldn't have known that I was looking at the pelvic region. According to the Ultrasound and MRI reports cancer hadn't been diagnosed yet. However, cancer couldn't be ruled out because my ovaries could not be visualized and the CA 125 was 50. This was elevated but it wasn't diagnostic. The normal value is 35 or less. The CT Scan wasn't scheduled until the 16th.

Finally I was next in line. A woman walked into the area and invited me to go into one of the offices. She said, "I'll be checking you in and verifying the accuracy of the information that we have. I'm also responsible for obtaining and logging in "co-pays" and referrals from your primary care physician. After we were done, I returned to the waiting area to wait to be called in.

Fortunately, I'd brought some reading with me. It not only seemed like a long wait. It was. When the nurse called me, she apologized, "It's been a really busy day today."

Gail took me into the clinic area and obtained my weight and blood pressure. My blood pressure was off the wall! She accompanied me into the examining area.

Immediately in front of me was a conference area: a round table and several chairs. To the right was the traditional examining area: examining table, wall oxygen and suction, and blood pressure apparatus and counter space, sink, and cabinets. Gail said, "Don't get undressed yet. Dr D likes to talk to you before you undress."

I sat in one chair and put my feet up on another, took out a journal from my backpack, and proceeded to read an article while I awaited her arrival. Although I appeared to be taking this in stride, I was nervous. On the one hand, I hoped that this would be a false alarm. On the other hand, I knew that I could have endometrial cancer or I could have myometrial cancer or I could have ovarian cancer. Inasmuch as the radiologists couldn't visualize my ovaries, I realized that ovarian cancer couldn't be ruled out.

When Dr. D came in to see me, I hastily put my journal aside and turned in my chair and put my feet on the floor. As I did, she extended her hand to me and greeted me. We shook hands. She had the reports that I had brought with me in her hands. She glanced at them briefly and looked at me. She asked, "Are you a nurse?"

"Yes."

Looking again at the notes, she commented, "This is very good."

I felt that I was still in control.

I didn't want to take any chances. I wanted her to have every piece of available information at her disposal. I'd written a summary letter of my trajectory to date and had attached the printed copies of my work-up.

Dr. D said, "I haven't looked at your films yet. Your CA 125 is elevated. As you know, it can be related to a number of things. Tell me, what happened at Dr. G's office."

I explained, "I was referred to him for an endometrial biopsy. He attempted the procedure but he couldn't insert the instrument. He said that he didn't want to risk perforating (puncturing) my uterus. He said that I had cancer and that you were the person whom I should see. I agree."

Dr. D said, "If he was unsuccessful, I'm not going to presume that I can succeed where he didn't. We can either take the slow road or the fast road. If we take the slow road, I would bring you in and do the procedure under anesthesia. Then we would talk about the next step. Or we could proceed directly to the surgery."

"I have a sizable fibroid and I'm going to need surgery. I would just as soon do that."

She said, "You are going to be scanned?"

I looked puzzled.

"CT Scan!"

"Oh, yes!" This was the first time that I realized that the CT Scan had a nickname.

My perception of the approaching surgery was a total abdominal hysterectomy and bilateral salpingo-oophorectomy (removal of womb, tubes, and ovaries). The surgery would involve tissue that was located in the pelvic cavity.

Following this discussion, Dr. D said, "I would like to examine you now. I will be back as soon as you are ready."

When she listened to my heart, she got really excited, "Wow, you have a systolic ejection murmur. Gail, listen to this! Is it okay if she listens? Has anyone told you that you have it?"

"Years ago, Dr. R told me that I had a physiologic murmur. Dr. T who is a cardiologist never told me that I had a murmur. I've only seen Dr. B once. She didn't say anything about a murmur."

During the vaginal examination, she sensed my discomfort during the opening of the speculum blades. She said, "I need to do a digital exam now. My fingers are very tiny." During the rectal examination, she commented, "You're already showing signs of obstruction."

When she was finished with the examination, she said, "You do need surgery. If you want me to do it, you'll probably need to come downtown." I was puzzled. I wondered, "Where was the downtown hospital? NSMC was in the next town."

"The only way that I could operate at NSMC is if I were to assist Dr. G. He doesn't do surgery anymore."

Suddenly, I realized that she was talking about the major teaching hospital *intown*. "Oh," I said, "I can go there."

She said, "I'm going to give you a card with the name and telephone number of the scheduling coordinator. If you want me to do the surgery, call her tomorrow to set up a time. Any questions?"

"Is it possible to do this surgery under epidural?" I knew instantly from her expression that she realized that I really didn't know that much about what was about to happen. She said, "You are afraid of anesthesia." I denied it, but I was afraid of everything. I knew that I needed surgery. I had committed to it.

She went on to tell me, "You need to talk with anesthesia. The epidural won't provide sufficient anesthesia during removal of the peritoneum (the lining of the abdominal cavity). I'd heard enough. I couldn't ask any more questions. I promised to call the next day and schedule the surgery.

This was Tuesday. I didn't call on Wednesday or Thursday. I planned to call Friday but I had the CT scan in the morning. I did remember to go to radiology to obtain the contrast material. The CT scan had been scheduled for 9:00 AM. The receptionist provided me with a plastic bottle containing 900 ml of contrast material, a ten-ounce cup, and instructions. My instructions were to eat nothing after 5:00 AM and to take 300 ml (10 ounces) of contrast material at 7:00 AM and at 7:30. I was to bring the remaining contrast material with me.

After signing in at ambulatory registration, I went to radiology. The receptionist took the remaining contrast material and I never saw it again. Although it wasn't as unpleasant as the drink that I had several years earlier, I wasn't anxious to drink any more. I was allowed to wear my own clothing.

The radiology technician escorted me into a small treatment area. After taking a brief history and verifying that I wasn't allergic to shellfish, she inserted an intravenous access line. An "iodine" contrast material is used during the CT Scan.

Then she and another technician escorted me into the procedure room. They assisted me onto the examining table and provided me with blankets, as the room was cold. From my perspective the procedure was very similar to the MRI without the "jackhammer."

The procedure is automated. The table is drawn into the large hollow tube and I am drawn in with it. The voice instructs me to take a deep breath and hold it as the table and I move outward. As instructed, I took deep breaths and held my breath in response to the computerized voice.

After several cycles of pictures, one of the technicians explained that she would now inject the "iodine". She told me that I would feel a warm sensation in the pelvic region. I did. I was drawn into the hollow tube, I attempted to coordinate taking deep breaths and holding breaths with the "voice" as the scanner did its work. As soon as the procedure was over, I was evicted from the hollow tube. The technicians assisted me off the table. After they explained how I would learn of the outcome, they sent me on my way.

Following the CT scan I went to work. I got held up in traffic on the way home from work. It was after five when I got home. I was distraught when I realized that I'd have to wait until Monday to call the scheduling coordinator. I would be thinking about this all weekend. I was upset that I had procrastinated earlier.

At 5:50 PM, the telephone rang. It was the scheduling coordinator. I was relieved to hear from her. I asked if I could wait until after the holidays.

She responded, "It's up to you. The first open date that I have is January 11th. We will let you know the time later. I will send you detailed instructions for your pre-op. You'll come in a few days before your surgery for blood work and a chest x-ray."

My primary care physician Dr B called me on November 17th to ask, "What is happening with the MRI and endometrial biopsy." I summarized what had been going on. After this conversation I e-mailed Dr D and mentioned Dr. B's call. I told her that I thought that Dr. B may have heard from the radiologist after the CT scan but she didn't say anything to indicate that she did or that any definitive findings were forthcoming. I shared my understanding of my situation with Dr D.

My perception was that I could have both endometrial cancer and ovarian cancer, either one or the other, or no cancer. If the latter turned out to be true, I would be delightfully surprised. At this time ovarian cancer hadn't been ruled out but no evidence that I had it had been forthcoming either. I realized that endometrial hyperplasia could be precancerous. Although I didn't mention it to her, I was concerned about the size of the fibroid and its growth rate.

The discomfort that I experienced when Dr. B examined me in January 2001 seemed to be in this area and it felt as if she were tugging on ligaments. Dr. B was now aware that I was scheduled for surgery on January 11th and agreed that it was the best way to proceed.

I went on to tell Dr. D that I did have more questions on the 13th but I couldn't handle any more information at the time. In this email I indicated that I was now ready for more information. I wanted to know how she would go about making the diagnosis, when would results of the biopsies be available, when would she start chemotherapy if it were indicated, and would I be able to donate blood in advance for use in surgery.

I obtained the films and a copy of the radiologist's report on November 19th. I looked at the films. As with the MRI, I wasn't successful in recognizing any normal anatomical structures in the pelvic region. I put the films aside. Later I looked at them again. The very last view on the very last film looked like a uterus—an anteverted uterus (i.e., bent forward). It appeared to be lit up—probably due to the contrast material. I also saw raggy-looking ureters (the tubes that drain urine from the kidneys to the bladder). They looked enormously dilated.

I left the CT scan films at the Cancer Center for Dr D the following day. I was overwhelmed. I thought, "If this is cancer, I'm going to die."

I was on a rapidly moving train that was heading somewhere that I didn't want to go. This was no ordinary train. It was the high-speed express train. On the one hand, the possibility of endometrial and/or ovarian cancer loomed overhead. On the other hand, it could be just a fibroid.

I fit the risk profile but the reports didn't confirm that I had either endometrial and/or ovarian cancer. I reasoned that the fibroid was a more likely cause of my symptoms. It didn't make sense that at my age the fibroid would be growing rather than shrinking.

The train was traveling at its highest speed and I didn't seem to be able to disembark.

2

People with Cancer Die

My early life experiences prior to my entry into nursing didn't expose me to people who had cancer and survived. They died. During my nursing career I didn't have a lot of experience caring for people with cancer. Most of them also died.

One of my earliest life experiences with cancer took place when I was in the ninth grade. Jim sat in the second row, third seat. I sat in the first row, second seat. Everyday from the first day of school through early November we talked about our life, our hopes, and our dreams. About homework, what we did over the weekend, the usual adolescent stuff. Jim was a bright boy and he was college bound. In early November Jim was absent for several days and we heard that he was very sick.

Nobody told us anything. In 1949 nobody would've told Jim anything either. He never returned to school. He must've suspected something. He was alive but not well at Christmas. No one broke the wall of silence to tell us whether Jim celebrated Christmas at home with his family or in the hospital. No one told us if he was well enough to know that it was Christmas. No one told us that Jim was going to die. On an unconscious level I knew it. Everyday I looked toward the third seat in the second row to see if Jim came back to school. He never did.

For the remainder of 1949 and for the beginning of 1950 his seat remained empty. If our homeroom teacher knew that Jim wasn't coming back to school, she never acknowledged it. She never assigned students who'd transferred into our school to his seat. His seat was empty in anticipation of his return.

One evening in February I was sitting at my desk doing my homework. I always had a lot of homework: Latin, English, history, social studies, and algebra. It was almost nine o'clock. The telephone rang. "Make it quick," my father called out, "It's almost nine o'clock." Making calls or answering the phone after nine o'clock was forbidden. This call was barely under the wire.

"Hello."

"Hi, this is Pat. Tim died. His funeral is tomorrow. Ask your parents if you can go."

"Tim? Do you mean Jim?" At that moment I realized that I knew all along that Jim was going to die.

"No, I mean Tim. He was sledding and he was run over by a truck."

Our class was in shock as we filed by his coffin in the funeral home overlooking the city common. Nothing in life had prepared us for losing a classmate. For many of us, including me, this was that first time that we had seen a dead person. None of us expected that the first dead person that we would see would be a young person—a classmate—someone our own age. For me, seeing him affirmed the reality of his death—not a reality that I wanted to face but one that I had to face.

The next day we returned to school and resumed our studies. We talked among ourselves but no one said anything to us. This is how it was in the 1950s.

Six days later, Pat called again. My worst fear was realized. Jim had died. I couldn't believe it. None of us had recovered from the shock of losing one classmate. Now we've lost another classmate. The following day we gathered for his funeral at the local Catholic Church. We weren't given the opportunity to see Jim. For me, not seeing him has resulted in his death seeming less real to me. As painful as it is to see the still, motionless body of a loved one, the day would come when I would realize how important it is.

Losing two classmates in less than one week was indescribably difficult. We never entertained the thought that we were vulnerable and that we could die. How did this happen? How did we lose two classmates in such a short time?

Somehow I came to know that Jim had cancer. In 1950 children with cancer died. Occasionally the local newspaper would feature an article about a child whose family was having Christmas in July for him or her. Having Christmas in July was a way of dealing with the reality of the impending death of a child who wouldn't live until Christmas. Having Christmas in July wasn't an option for Jim's family. If it had been, Jim certainly would have known that something was amiss.

This was my first encounter with cancer. My friend died.

Five years later I was a student at a small college on the Fenway. I worked part time as a nursing assistant at a nearby teaching hospital. Faith, a twenty-three-year old, woman with lymphoma was admitted in spring 1955. No one ever told me that Faith had lymphoma. Inadvertently I overheard report one day and learned this. For the longest time I didn't know whether Faith knew that she had cancer. In 1955 no one told cancer patients that they had cancer.

Faith had worked for an insurance company in town. She spoke of her job and her experiences. She would recite a rhyme that explained the meaning of the weather lights on its tower.

> *Steady blue—clear view*
> *Flashing blue—clouds due*
> *Steady red—rain ahead*
> *Flashing red—snow instead*

Sometimes she used the words of the rhyme to describe the kind of day she expected to have. I knew that she expected a really bad day if she said, "Flashing red!" I hoped for but never heard her say, "Steady blue!"

Caring for Faith was a challenge. She was easily fatigued and often couldn't tolerate essential care. I was usually assigned to provide her with basic physical care—bathing her and changing her bed linens. Frequently she asked me to provide her care immediately so that she can rest or to delay her care while she rested. For several weeks I was able to adapt my schedule to meet her needs and to keep her as comfortable as reasonably possible.

One day while I was bathing her, Faith told me, "I know that I have cancer." I looked into her eyes, but I said nothing.

She continued, "When you wake up day after day feeling sick and not getting any better, you figure it out."

Sadly, I wasn't in a position to confirm or deny that she had cancer. However, I could be flexible and adapt my schedule to her fatigue level and make her as comfortable as possible.

In July I had an unexpected luxury of having only two patients to care for. Unfortunately I was working under the direction of a nursing student who was learning to manage patient care. The student told me to bath Ms. C who had a heart problem first, as she was my sickest patient and then to bathe Faith who wasn't as sick.

After breakfast I went into Ms. C's cubicle. Ms. C said, "I'm really tired from eating. Could I rest for a half-hour before you bathed me?" A few minutes later Faith asked me, "Can you bathe me now so I can take a nap?" Never in my wildest dreams did I think that adapting my schedule to meet the needs of both women would create havoc.

The next day my supervisors took me aside and reprimanded me for not following the directions of the nursing student. I tried to explain to them that I was responding to the expressed wishes of both patients but they refused to listen to me. What dismays me most about this situation is that if I had done as directed both patients would've been worse off. On this day I had the luxury of being assigned to provide basic care to two women. I could respond to their requests and meet their expressed needs.

On other occasions I had been assigned to provide basic care to ten patients all of whom were sicker that either of these women to whom I had been assigned on this particular day. Shortly after this incident I left my position at this teaching hospital and took a position in a hospital in my hometown.

Several weeks later I learned that Faith had died. This was my second encounter with cancer. My former patient had died.

Meanwhile in my hometown hospital the maternity supervisor recruited me to work on the maternity unit. I worked there until I entered my basic nursing program at the hospital.

While I was a nursing student, I cared for many patients with cancer. I recall some with whom I had extended contact. One of my patients was a former third grade classmate. After being held back a few times, she left school at age sixteen. When we were 22 she had her seventh child. Now at age 25 she had extensive surgery for vaginal cancer—the excised area was left open to heal on its own. She died shortly after I cared for her.

As a first year nursing student I scrubbed in on a case in which the woman had extensive metastases throughout her abdomen. The entire abdominal wall was involved. I touched her cancer. That evening I worked on the unit where she and the other patients for whom I had scrubbed that day in surgery were recovering from their surgery. I witnessed the impact of her surgery on her life. Within a few weeks she died.

The commonly expressed lay theory or old wives' tale at this time was, "if they open you up and air gets to the cancer, that's it, there's no hope, death is certain." People in the 1960s weren't aware that death would've been more likely at a time in history when late diagnosis occurred and a paucity of treatment options was available.

As a senior nursing student I was assigned to the night shift. During the early 1960s cardiopulmonary resuscitation response teams and intensive care units had not yet come into being. Nursing students were in charge of patient care units and worked under the supervision of a nursing supervisor who was responsible for several units. In this hospital one supervisor covered the front of the house and another covered the back of the house. The unit to which I had been assigned was in the back of the house. It had previously been the children's unit.

The unit had a two-bed room at its entrance around the corner from the nurses' station, a two-bed room across from the nurses' station, a three-bed room next to the nurses' station. The corridor led into a large open ward with eight beds—four on the left and four on the right. The large ward opened into a solarium that had been converted into a three-bed room.

I arrived at 11:00 PM and listened to report. Most of the patients on the unit were stable and were recovering. One patient had had major abdominal surgery and was very unstable. After report the evening nurse and I made rounds. All beds on the unit except three were occupied. As we entered the large open ward, the curtains were drawn in front of the four beds on the left. Three of the four beds on the left were unoccupied. Only the third bed on the left was occupied.

When we entered the large ward, the evening nurse entered the curtained off area on the left between the first and second cubicle and made her way to the third cubicle. I followed her. We assessed the woman's status. It was grave. She was lying on her right side. Oxygen was flowing through a tube into her right nostril. . Stomach contents were being drawn through a tube in her left nostril into a collecting receptacle. Intravenous fluid was flowing through a tube into her left arm. The dressing on her abdomen was bulky and dry. Dark urine was dripping very slowly from a tube that emptied into a bag that was hooked on her bed. Her face had a bluish yellow tinge. She was barely responsive. Her blood pressure was very low.

As we assessed her condition, the resident entered the cubicle. He reviewed the orders that he had written. He had left specific guidelines for when to call him. He instructed me, "If her condition changes—if you notice any of these changes, call me directly. I will be at this extension."

At least three times I called him. He responded promptly and worked vigorously to stabilize her. I followed his directions precisely. Then he returned to the on-call room. The on-call room was the designated place where the residents could sleep in between calls to the units for urgent changes in patient conditions.

When the nursing supervisor made rounds, I updated her on the woman's status. She berated me for violating hospital policy by calling the resident without notifying her first. She admonished me to call her the next time I observed a change in the woman's status. When the woman's condition deteriorated again, I called the nursing supervisor. She came promptly and assessed her status. She called the resident but the woman died before the resident arrived. The resident was distraught. He had tried so hard and now he could do no more.

The supervisor explained to the resident, "I instructed her to call me. I'm sorry." The resident noted on her death certificate that the cause of death was carcinoma of the pancreas. This information wasn't reported to me earlier.

In spite of the fact that the prognosis for carcinoma of the pancreas in the 1963s was very poor, the resident had invested a great deal of energy into her care. Much of my time had also been invested in her care. Fortunately, few patients had medications scheduled during the night and the nursing assistant was able to do vital signs and meet the personal hygiene needs of the remaining patients.

After her death, I made rounds to assess the conditions of my remaining patients. Everyone was stable. I thought that everyone in the beds on the right side of the ward were asleep. We didn't want to disturb their sleep.

When the woman's son came in to see his mother for the last time, he whispered, "Thank you." I responded, "I'm so sorry!" After he left, we made every effort to move her from the ward to the morgue without letting the other patients know what was happening. This is how it was in the 1960s.

Several hours later, the day staff arrived, listened to report, and went to work. They quietly opened the curtains that had been closed since the woman had returned from surgery. The day had begun.

The night had ended for me. I went to breakfast and went back to the nurses' residence to go to sleep. The impact of the night was definitely not over.

The following week I was assigned to the day shift. One of my patients was agitated but I didn't know what to do. I had no idea what was wrong. I could do nothing to meet her needs. In frustration, I said, "If you don't tell me what is wrong, I can't help you." She sobbed inconsolably, "You didn't know it but I was awake the night the woman died. You looked in on me and I pretended to be asleep but I was awake. I knew everything that was going on."

"I'm so sorry," I responded. "I didn't know."

At that moment I knew that the way that we were dealing with death wasn't right but I didn't know what we should be doing.

I didn't realize that my concept of cancer as a terminal disease was being formed. My early exposure to persons with cancer featured death as an inevitable outcome. Most of my life's work as a nurse has been in Maternal and Child

Health clinical and educational settings. I rarely encountered patients who had cancer.

Suddenly I was on a high-speed train and I didn't want to take the journey. The destination was death! I'd been so cool when I went to see Dr. D. I had the paperwork and the films in order. She could look it over. She could examine me. She could tell me that I didn't have cancer.

It didn't go that smoothly. Dr. D read the reports. She examined me. She said that she couldn't tell me that I didn't have cancer. Nor could she tell me that I did. She could tell me how she would go about finding out the answer. She did.

I wasn't anxious to cross over—to become a patient. The whole world looks so different when it becomes a *View from the Other Side of the Looking Glass.*

3

Coming out of the Dark Tunnel

If you want to see clearly in a dark tunnel, you need to close your eyes briefly. Your pupils will enlarge and allow more light to enter. Then you can see more clearly. Everything was so blurry. I must have forgotten to close my eyes.

The high-speed express train on which I was traveling was being propelled full speed ahead through a very dark tunnel. The barely perceptible sights that moved into and out of my line of vision were frightening. Most of the lights on the train were off. During my journey through the dark tunnel I'd only seen glimpses of the past that had yielded devastating results. Finally a glimmer of light began to appear.

My perspective began to change. On November 24th I dared to ask Dr. D more questions. I e-mailed a list of questions to her. Her downtown nurse Joanna called with answers to my questions. Pathologists would be standing by to examine the tissue samples and lymph nodes as soon as they were removed from my body and tentative results would be provided. Final results wouldn't be available until the following week. If chemotherapy were indicated, I would receive the first doses prior to leaving the hospital after surgery. Sufficient bleeding to warrant transfusion wasn't likely. Donating blood in advance for use in surgery didn't seem necessary. The catheter in my bladder would be removed the next day. As soon as I was passing gas and eating food, the intravenous tube in my arm would be removed. I knew all this. This is standard practice. But I had to ask. I needed to know if this was really happening to me. I was taking a tiny peek—trying to see the *View from the Other Side of the Looking Glass*. I didn't linger on the other side for very long.

In December my brother spent a weekend in New Hampshire taking antacids. He believed that he had indigestion. On Monday he called his health care provider and made an appointment. He left work early and drove himself to his appointment. The physician who saw him made arrangements for him to be transferred to a North Shore Hospital by ambulance where he was admitted to the coronary care unit. Fortunately his heart attack was mild. I became the baby sitter for my niece and nephew so that his wife could be at his side.

When I went to visit him the next following day, he'd been transferred to a step-down unit where he began cardiac rehabilitation. An interdisciplinary team comprised of a nurse, dietician, physical therapist, and occupational therapist provided teaching and set his rehabilitation plan into motion. Prior to his discharge he underwent cardiac catheterization at the North Shore Hospital. He was then transferred to a major teaching hospital in Boston where he had a stent inserted into a heart vessel. Afterwards he was discharged home where he continued his rehabilitation. In the meantime my journey continued.

As the high speed express train moved out of the dark tunnel into the daylight, I tried to make sense of the journey. Unexpectedly in December I began to have recurrent symptoms. I kept a log of every symptom and sensation that I experienced. I was sure that Dr. D would need this information to make a diagnosis. I tried to make sense of my symptoms and arrive at my own diagnosis. This wouldn't be easy. I tried to determine my treatment regimen. In the meantime I began to feel more optimistic about my future. I made definite plans.

I knew that I couldn't have dental work during chemotherapy. Instead of waiting until January I scheduled a second gum graft with the periodontist in early December. This graft went more smoothly than an earlier one. I used relaxation breathing throughout the procedure and almost fell asleep. My recovery was uneventful.

The recurrent symptoms and sensations were annoying. The periodic onset of premenstrual-like symptoms and pelvic congestion was followed by approximately 4–5 ml (a teaspoon) of bright bleeding. The intervals between each episode decreased from seven to six to five to four days.

The worst episode occurred on Christmas Day. Initially I had been reluctant to have surgery before the holiday. I'd been recoiling from the potential cancer diagnosis and the possibility that this would be my last Christmas. We spent the day with the family at my brother's home. He and his wife are raising their grandchildren. Their oldest daughter, the children's mother had been killed in an automobile crash. Their younger daughter and her husband and their son and his future fiancée joined us for the festivities.

We had a great time watching the children open their gifts—toys and games and new clothes. We enjoyed a delightful meal and playing with the new games. Their daughter and her husband and their son and his future fiancée went home around 5:00 PM. The children took their stuff to their rooms and were playing quietly upstairs. We were having wine or coffee and dessert.

Suddenly I experienced a gush of bleeding. I asked to be excused and I headed upstairs. As I arrived at the top of the stairs, my niece asked, "Auntie, can you help me open my music box?"

I said, "I will after I go to the bathroom." I returned and I helped her.

After she played the music box, she asked, "Will you read me a story?"

I had another gush of bleeding. I said, "I need to go to the bathroom."

She looked puzzled. "But, Auntie, you just went."

"I know."

A few minutes later, I returned and said, "Great Grammy and I need to go home now. Why don't you come down stairs and say 'goodbye' to her?"

I hastily made plans to leave. I was home within a few minutes. I didn't know how long this bleeding would persist. I didn't lock the door as I thought that I might have to call 911.

These episodes greatly alarmed me. I tried to think clearly. "What do I do now? If I call 911, will they take me to the local hospital or will I be able to persuade them to take me to the hospital where my downtown doctor practices? What if they decide that I don't have cancer and won't refer me to my downtown doctor for surgery? What if my downtown doctor isn't on call and they can't reach her and what if…?"

As these thoughts ran wildly through my head, I began to realize that the bleeding was subsiding. I'd seen another *View from the Other Side of the Looking Glass*. Now, I could return to the more familiar side. I could be the nurse and watch and wait.

I called Dr D's downtown office the day after Christmas. Dr D was away. Her nurse Joanna was available.

Joanna asked, "What is your diagnosis?"

I hesitated as I was being bombarded with the overwhelming load of information that I'd been accumulating since November. I didn't actually know my diagnosis. I had a few "could be this" diagnoses and a "hope it is this" diagnosis. It was like a multiple-choice test question with several answers, including options of "all of these" or "none of these."

During my search of my various textbooks and journals and the Internet, I had become aware that multiple possibilities existed. I wasn't at high risk for some gynecologic cancers and I was at high risk for others.

Some gynecologic cancers, such as vaginal, and cervical, are related to human papilloma virus—a sexually transmitted disease. Inasmuch as I hadn't been sexually active, I didn't consider myself a risk for these cancers. Vaginal cancer accounts for 1–2% of gynecologic cancers. Abnormal vaginal bleeding is the most common symptom associated with vaginal cancer. Watery discharge and painful intercourse may be present. Cervical cancer accounts for 6% of cancer that affects women. It's the third most common gynecologic cancer. Bleeding after intercourse and between menstrual periods is typical. Early age at first intercourse and multiple partners increases risk.

Other gynecologic cancers, such as uterine cancers and ovarian cancers have a different set of associated risk factors. I soon became aware that I was at risk for these cancers. As the fourth most common cancer in women and the most common gynecologic cancer, endometrial cancer (one form of uterine cancer) accounts for 13% of malignancies affecting women. Endometrial cancer is usually diagnosed at an early stage and it has a five-year survival rate of 85%. Ovarian cancers are the second most common group of gynecologic cancers and account for a greater percent of mortality than all other gynecologic malignancies combined. Ovarian cancers are usually diagnosed during the later stages and have a five-year survival rate of 20%.

Obesity is the most significant risk factor for endometrial cancer (cancer of the inner lining of the uterus or womb). Nulliparity (having never borne children), late menopause and unopposed estrogen are also risk factors. Endometrial hyperplasia often precedes endometrial cancer. Abnormal post-menopausal uterine bleeding often accompanies endometrial cancer. Endometrial biopsy or sampling of the lining of the uterus is usually done in the gynecologist's office to detect endometrial cancer.

Ironically ovarian cancer and endometrial cancer shared some of the same risks: obesity, absence of childbearing and late menopause. However, abnormal postmenopausal uterine bleeding was an unlikely sign in ovarian cancer. Endometrial cancer and ovarian cancer were very real possibilities; the possibility that I had a leiomyoma (fibroid) had not been ruled out. I knew that a suspected leiomyoma could be a sarcoma. I still wanted to cast my vote for a fibroid!

Obesity, absence of childbearing, late menopause, and now abnormal post-menopausal uterine bleeding were part of my presenting history. The reports of the diagnostic tests provided additional data but no definitive answer.

The transabdominal and intervaginal ultrasound reports indicated two findings: 1. Thickening of the endometrium that *could be* hyperplasia, polyp, or neoplasm, and 2. Solid mass (8.3 x 9.0 cm.) adjacent to the lateral border of the uterus that *could be* a broad ligament myoma. Neither ovary could be visualized. In my case, had the biopsy attempted as an office procedure been successful, it might've contributed to the differential diagnosis of the endometrial changes. The biopsy wouldn't have clarified the status of the prominent solid mass or the elusive ovaries.

The major focus of the MRI was to differentiate between ovarian neoplasm and broad ligament myoma. The mass measures 9.4 x 8.9 x 6.3 cm. Although the images supported the diagnosis of leiomyoma, the ovaries couldn't be definitively identified. In addition, the CT Scan confirmed the presence of pelvic mass measuring 10 cm. x 6.5 cm. x 10 cm. that could be of uterine or ovarian origin. Once again the ovaries couldn't be visualized.

I was trying to sort out what I knew from what I wanted to believe as I fumbled for an answer to Joanna's question. I finally said, "I don't know. I could have endometrial or ovarian cancer but maybe I have a fibroid."

After listening to my description of my symptoms, Joanna said, "I think that it is probably the fibroid. How bad is it (the bleeding) now?"

I answered, "It's stopped."

She asked, "Who's assisting Dr. D?"

I responded, "I don't know. She's doing the surgery intown because the gynecologist I went to doesn't operate anymore. I have no idea who'll be assisting her."

Joanna went on to say, "Dr. D is away for the rest of the week. If you start to bleed again, call me right away. If nothing happens, call me Friday anyway. I want to be sure that you are okay going into the weekend."

The rest of the week was uneventful. I spoke with Joanna on Friday and told her that everything seemed to be under control. That evening I had minor spotting and wasn't alarmed.

As I continued on this fast moving train, I realized that I wouldn't escape unscathed by cancer. I just didn't know what its name would be. I had a collection of books that I kept turning to—looking for explanations. The ones that I found most helpful were The Merck Manual of Diagnosis and Therapy, 17th edition, edited by Mark H. Beers and Robert Berkow and Everyone's Guide to Cancer Therapy, 3rd edition, by Malin Dollinger, Ernest H. Rosenbaum, and Greg Cable. The latter book is now in its fourth edition.

I tried to guess what course of treatment I could expect. As I read, I found that discussion of types of gynecologic cancer other than ovarian cancer were easier to understand than discourse about the various types of ovarian cancer. I tried to avoid thinking about the likelihood that I had ovarian cancer.

Uterine cancers could involve the endothelium or lining, the muscle layer, or the cervix or opening of the uterus. If I had uterine cancer, I suspected that I probably had endometrial cancer. The definitive statements in the radiologists' reports helped me keep this potential outcome in perspective and supported my conclusion.

Ovarian cancers could involve the epithelium or outer surface of the ovary or supportive tissues or the ova (eggs). According to the radiologists' reports, my ovaries couldn't be visualized. I decided that if I had ovarian cancer I probably had one of the more aggressive, rapidly growing cancers of the germ cells or ova—probably a teratoma. The radiologists didn't provide any reassuring statements that would lessen my emerging worries about the worst possible scenario.

The smorgasbord of ovarian cancers and the variety of treatment protocols made it difficult for me to reach any firm conclusions about the course of treatment at this time. However I realized that carboplatin (Paraplatin) and paclitaxel (Taxol) were likely candidates for chemotherapy.

In two weeks I would have surgery and the truth would be known. In the meantime I plunged myself into my work. As a nursing faculty member, I had primary responsibility for two major courses. I planned to return to work second semester. I knew that I had to have a plan in place in case everything didn't go as planned and I developed a plan.

As a nurse I knew that much of my recovery depended on my ability to mobilize myself after surgery. I set a plan in motion to achieve mobility and optimum recovery. I'd observed the differences between the achieved outcomes of Amy's firm but gentle approach with the maternity patients after cesarean birth and the unachieved outcomes of other nurses' laissez faire approaches with similar patients. I was determined to use Amy's approach as a model for my recovery.

I'd been getting up so frequently during the night that I had no need to roll over in bed. I wondered if I would be able to roll from side to side in bed to get into a comfortable position. I'd watched young women who were a little overweight struggle to sit up and stand prior to walking. I knew that I needed to get up and walk if I expected my body to recover from surgery. I exercised to strengthen the muscles that I would use to achieve these goals. In spite of my growing fatigue as the day for surgery approached, I conscientiously exercised.

Finally the time for surgery arrived.

4

Uprooting the Enemy

During the days preceding my upcoming surgery on January 11, 2002 the high speed express train really sped up—as if it weren't going fast already. I had lunch with a good friend on Tuesday. Lunch with Mary is always an invigorating experience.

Sometimes we are reminded of *The Strange World of Mr. Mum*—a comic strip that used to be featured in the Boston Sunday Globe. As Mr. Mum contemplated the strange events that were taking place around him, he wondered why others didn't realize that things that perplexed him were strange. Often Mary and I discussed circumstances that perplexed us and wondered why others weren't troubled about them.

Today was no different. We discussed life's problems and proposed reasonable solutions. We also discussed my upcoming surgery. Although Mary never had cancer, she had the primary surgery I was about to have. The surgery had improved her quality of life. This, of course, was welcome news to me.

On Wednesday I'd been scheduled for the Pre-Test Day. The Pre-Test Day was scheduled two days prior to Same Day Admission for surgery to ensure that data essential for surgery was obtained and specific tests were performed. The results inform the surgeon and the anesthesiologist of problems that need to be corrected prior to or addressed during anesthesia and surgery.

I arrived as scheduled for what could be a three-hour tour somewhat reminiscent of Gilligan's Island. I was supposed to go to radiology at 12:30 PM for a chest x-ray and then to general admitting for other preoperative work.

I entered the primary reception area of the hospital and followed the signs to General Admitting. I had to stop at the Rest Room on the way. When I arrived, I glanced at my instructions and realized that I should've gone to Radiology first. I returned to the primary reception area. On the way I made another stop at the Rest Room. The reception area at radiology was under construction so I followed directions and found the temporary reception desk. I didn't have a blue card so I had to retrace my steps to an office near the General Admitting Area. I was already exhausted and the fun hadn't even begun. The woman at the "Blue Card Office" was both compassionate and competent. She assured me that if I lost this one I could get another by calling in.

I trudged back to Radiology, checked in, and joined the large crowd that was waiting for pictures of various sorts. The wait wasn't long but the intervals between my need for a Rest Room were short. After I posed for a chest x-ray I found the stairwell and the corridor that would take me back to General Admitting. When I saw a yellow (closed for cleaning) sign outside of the next Rest Room, I groaned. I found another one just in time.

The receptionist at General Admitting told me that I had to go to see the surgeon who would be performing the surgery. Her office was in a building some distance away. When I arrived I saw the sign that indicated that this building was the Cancer Center. I asked myself, "What am I doing here? I don't have cancer." Actually deep down inside I knew that I did. I kept that knowledge buried deep down inside so that it couldn't escape and taunt me.

The receptionist in the Cancer Center called the surgeon's assistant and said, "Dr. D's 11:00 o'clock is here. I was surprised. I thought out loud, "No one told me that I had an 11:00 o'clock appointment." The receptionist said, "Someone may have written your name there so that we would fit you in."

Dr. D's assistant escorted me into an exam room and told me to sit in a chair. Several minutes later Dr. D burst into the exam room and knelt quickly on the floor in front of me. She was wearing a white coat. She placed the consent forms on the physician's stool and explained the surgery to me. The form indicated that Dr D would perform a total abdominal hysterectomy (TAH), bilateral salpingo-oophorectomy (BSO), remove a pelvic mass and take biopsies of several lymph nodes. I would later learn that the pathologist measured the left adnexal mass as it was called preoperatively at 14 cm (5 ½ inches) by 9 cm (3 ½ inches) by 9 cm (3

½ inches). I knew that Dr. D would be removing a lot of tissue but I didn't hesitate one second. I promptly signed the surgical consent form. This surgery was inevitable. Another visit to the Rest Room was pending.

After I signed the consent, Dr. D said, "Now that I am down here, I hope that I can get up."

Since she looked quite agile when she entered, I retorted, "I'm sure that you can get up quicker than I can. I'm not moving too fast these days"

She announced something that I hadn't observed earlier, "This baby is really anxious to get out of here."

"How long do you have?" I asked.

She replied, "Four weeks. You probably got in under the wire. I don't know how much longer I'll be able to operate." Then she asked, "Do you have any questions?"

I commented, "I know about the surgery. The only thing that puzzles me is that I don't understand how I can have a problem related to too much estrogen [endometrial hyperplasia] and a problem related to too little estrogen [osteoporosis] at the same time.

Dr D responded, "Not all cancer is caused by estrogen."

Her answer puzzled me but I was in denial at the moment about the possibility of cancer. Moreover, it contradicted my theory.

Before I left, Dr D explained, "I may see you late Friday afternoon if you are awake. If not, I will see you Saturday morning."

I continued my journey. Finally I arrived at General Admitting for the last time, showed the receptionist my Blue Card and insurance cards, and gave her other routine information—who I was, whom to notify, No, I didn't have a Health Care Proxy, Yes, I had that information, etc. She asked me to sign a consent form. I did. I didn't want to spend the rest of my life visiting the Rest Room.

The receptionist also gave me several forms to complete. She asked me to answer a nutrition questionnaire, which I did. While I was completing the forms, a nurse in a white coat entered the waiting area and called my name.

After introducing herself, she explained that she was a research coordinator. She explained, "If you're willing to take part in this study, some of the tissue that would be removed during surgery, some blood samples, and some of the urine that would be collected during the surgery would be used."

Being a research participant wasn't new to me. I was already a participant in the Nurses' Health Study. Every other day I take low dose aspirin or placebo and vitamin E or placebo. The study that I was being invited to take part in would provide important information for Women's Health. I had no desire to take my tumor home in a bottle! I planned to participate.

Reviewing the proposal and the consent form in the waiting area was a weird experience. Focusing on the pages in front of me was tough. I knew what it should say. I wanted to be sure it did. Every crowd has its wise guy! The wise guy in this crowd said, "Be careful. They aren't telling you that they're going to take the tissue sample from your left big toe!" I tried not to laugh too hard.

I looked at the research coordinator and said, "I'm going to sign this. I just want to be a responsible participant and read the consent form thoroughly to be sure that my rights are protected." Nonetheless I wasn't reading it from a patient's perspective.

I read that the study was designed to detect markers of ovarian cancer and that my participation in this study didn't mean that I had ovarian cancer. When I read this, I thought to myself, "They need people who don't have ovarian cancer to be in the control group." Denial does wonders! I signed the consent form and returned the papers to the research coordinator. She gave me several blood tubes and asked me to give them to the technician who would be doing my preoperative work-up.

A short time later a medical technician called me. After weighing me, she checked my vital signs (blood pressure, temperature, heart rate, and breathing rate) and performed an electrocardiogram. Then she took blood from a vein in my arm and instructed me to provide a urine specimen.

After the tests were completed, I joined the rapidly expanding crowd in another waiting area. Soon a nurse called my name and led me to a room where the teaching would take place. When she learned that I was a nurse, she didn't spend much time explaining what she perceived that I would know. However, she emphasized several important points. She pointed out the importance of deep breathing exercises to prevent postoperative pneumonia and explained the importance of measures to prevent deep vein clots that could break away and block major blood vessels. For the former, I would be given a gadget that would promote lung expansion. For the latter, I would be given elastic stockings and would be provided with compression boots that would facilitate circulation. Although she never mentioned that a catheter would be placed in my bladder, I knew that this would take place. I just didn't know when.

The next person to see me was the anesthesiologist who asked me a lot of questions about my medical history and informed me that I would be put to sleep during the surgery. I had sorted of hoped that I would be a participant observer. I was never clear how I would actually take part in the surgery but I did seem to think that somehow I would be able to see what was going on. For some reason he left the room for a moment. When he returned, he said, "I think that we will be putting you to sleep!" My preoperative visit was over. After a facility visit I headed home. The good news was that I had no problems that would interfere with my upcoming surgery. My surgeon and her team would be able to attack the eggplant-sized tumor as scheduled.

The next day my Annual Physical Examination with my Primary Care Physician was scheduled. This was my second visit with her. I'd already visited a GYN Oncologist twice, once more than I had visited my latest Primary Care Physician.

As the day for my surgery approached I became more acutely aware of an issue that I had tended to brush aside. I had bravely stepped up to the plate when I visited Dr. D in November and stated bravely, "Take it all out. I'm not going to Italy for fertility treatment at my age."

As a consequence of this surgery I was about to be deprived of my womanhood! My ovaries—the hallmark of femininity and the source of estrogen—were about to be excised. As I had sought answers to my questions—one being how could I have a cancer that was related to too much estrogen and osteoporosis that was related to too little estrogen—I was reminded that the ovaries aren't the body's only source of estrogen. The ovary secretes estrogen in harmony with the ovulation process. However, a more common source of most estrogen or estrone in children, men, and women who are postmenopausal or who do not ovulate exists. Estrone results from synthesis of a steroid produced by the adrenal gland (a gland that lies over the kidneys) and takes place in adipose tissue.

I always thought that in spite of my postmenopausal status I had an abundance of estrogen. Physiologic changes that generally accompany menopause didn't seem to affect me as they did other women. Tissue that normally shrunk during menopause hadn't shrunk and hair that normally thinned out hadn't thinned out.

When I had visited my new Primary Care Physician for the first time one year ago, she had recommended a cholesterol panel, a bone density test, and a sigmoidoscopy.

When she sent me the results of my cholesterol panel last year, I was alarmed. My total cholesterol had risen. I always got mixed up on which cholesterol was the good cholesterol and which was the bad cholesterol.

I set out to reverse this unexpected derangement with no holds barred. This attack involved changes in my diet that resulted in a more heart friendly diet: reduced fat (from > 30% to < 27%) and reduced cholesterol (from > 10% to < 7%>). I did not look at the number of total calories as I had done in the past because this approach had not worked for me before. The results were surprisingly delightful. For the first time since excess weight had become a problem, I began to lose weight at a slow, steady pace.

In the past I had tried weight watchers and had lost weight. Unfortunately, I regained it. I had also focused on reducing total caloric intake. Initially I lost a few pounds but this trend would reverse itself. I would gain weight and become discouraged.

Later I realized that although the total cholesterol had been elevated, the bad cholesterol had gone down and the good cholesterol had gone up. I could never remember which was the good and which was the bad. I made up this little jingle. "When your low is high and your high is low; you haven't gone very far to go!"

When my primary care physician had informed me in spring 2001 that I had osteoporosis, she discussed the options with me. I was adamant that I did not want to take estrogen. After I researched alendronate on the Internet and discussed it with a former RN student who had called me for something else, I agreed to take the weekly therapeutic dose.

While I was looking for answers to my current pressing medical problem (the left adnexal mass or tumor, elevated CA 125, and thickened endometrial stripe), I learned that the body uses cholesterol during the synthesis of estrogen. I wondered if I had foiled the enemy by depriving it of one of its basic necessities when I cut back on the bad cholesterol. Later I read that estrogen is supposed to promote the good cholesterol.

After verifying that I was here for my second Annual Physical Examination with her, my Primary Care Physician decided to listen to my heart and lungs to be sure that I was okay for anesthesia. She explained that it was too early to do a follow-up bone density examination.

Then she said, "You should have a colonoscopy!"

I commented, "You had suggested a sigmoidoscopy last year but I wasn't brave enough then."

She said no more about it.

I asked, "Should I speak with your nurse about scheduling it?"

She said, "Oh, I wasn't sure that you were going to do it."

I responded, "Well, I don't want to but I will."

I was thinking, "Last year, she was talking about a procedure that involved a small portion of the end of the bowel. Now, she is talking about a procedure that involves the entire bowel. I had better sign on before she expands her request again." Mary had already told me that the latter procedure was no picnic!"

She explained the scheduling process. She also completed a referral for the surgery in case one had not been faxed to the hospital where the surgery would take place.

The woman who does colonoscopy scheduling told me that the earliest opening was in early June. This was okay with me. I wasn't eager to have the procedure. Later she called me and rescheduled the procedure on July 3rd. At the time, I thought, "This is even better. I am in no hurry."

Following the visit to my Primary Care Physician I went to my office and verified that everything that I would need for the first day of class was assembled. After making certain that I could breeze into the office on the first day of class and pick everything that I needed, I went home to prepare for the next day.

Actually the prep had started two weeks earlier as I wasn't allowed to take aspirin or ibuprofen or any products containing either for two weeks prior to the surgery. Not taking these medications prior to surgery is important as they impede clotting and may result in undesired bleeding during and after surgery.

I didn't know it at the time, but I had the "easy prep." At four o'clock I drank eight ounces of Citrate of Magnesia. After a light supper, I couldn't eat nor could I drink anything after midnight. I had been instructed to use a Fleet Enema on the morning of surgery. Citrate of Magnesia is very effective. The enema didn't seem to be necessary. However, the teaching form points out that surgery could be cancelled if the instructions aren't followed. I did what I could to follow the instructions to the letter of the law. I didn't like traveling on the high-speed express train but I didn't want to jump off while it was in motion.

January 11th, the day that my surgery was scheduled, had arrived. My years at Children's Rehabilitation Center had serendipitously rewarded me with a familiarity with the morning traffic patterns around the hospital. I told my brother that if he picked me up at 6:15 AM, we would be there on time.

My bags had been packed earlier that week. In spite or the fact that I was not a morning person, I was ready to roll when he came by to drive me to the hospital. Nothing was going to interfere with my pending surgery that would free me from my dependence of the facilities.

He drove into the hospital complex and left me off at the revolving door. I made my way to the Same Day Surgery Reception Area. A few minutes after I reported in, a nursing assistant called me into the change area and gave me hospital gown, trousers, robe, elastic stockings, nonskid slippers, a huge white bag for my clothing and duffel bag, and a stringed tag with my name and hospital record number. I removed almost everything and stepped into my non-glamorous outfit.

I surrendered all of my personal possessions—everything but a deck of cards. I had too much money with me but they had already taken it for safekeeping. I sat in the waiting area and I waited. In an adjoining room children were waiting with their parents for surgery. I thought, "If kids can do this, I should be able to."

A woman called me and led me into a room. I saw the electronic blood pressure monitoring equipment and prepared to have my blood pressure checked.

The woman said, "Oh, I'm not the nurse. You said that you wanted to see a priest but the priest isn't here today. He asked me to fill in for him. We all believe in the same God. If it's okay, I can pray with you." I never refuse offers of prayers. I believe that her prayers helped.

Again I waited in the waiting area for the nurse. I was called in again. I got ready to have my blood pressure checked. She attached a cuff to my arm and pressed the right button. The cuff got really tight. I could feel a cable tightening on my arm.

I protested, "This is too tight."

She said, "They get really tight."

I repeated, "No, this is much too tight."

The digital readout for my blood pressure was "241/247!"

I commented wryly, "The first number is lower than the second number. That should be your first clue that the reading is wrong. Check it again."

The second reading was somewhat elevated but within a more acceptable range. My surgery could proceed.

Again I was told to wait in the waiting area. I was called one last time. A woman led me to the surgical suite. I hesitated as we passed the last Rest Room on the way to the surgical suite. The woman asked, "Do you want to make a stop?"

I responded, "I guess not. I should be okay. They will be putting a catheter in any minute." Later I would wish that I had made one last stop.

The woman brought me to stretcher 29 and notified an orderly that I'd arrived. He introduced himself, "I am Luis, your orderly for the day. When it's time for you to go to surgery, I'll be taking you to operating room 29 where you'll have your operation."

A nurse approached and said, "I have heparin for you."

I started to lift my hospital gown to bare my abdomen.

She said, "I need to give it in your arm. I can't inject heparin into your abdomen today because you're having surgery there."

Shortly thereafter Luis transported me to pre-anesthesia room 29 and told me, "It won't be long now. Your nurse will be right in."

A few minutes later, Lori, my primary nurse, arrived. After introducing herself, she verified information that was on the medical record and asked other questions. She asked, "Are you anxious? I nodded. She told me, "Dr D is my doctor. She is really good. When the nurses go to your doctor, you know that your doctor is good."

She mentioned that she had graduated from the nursing education program at North Shore Community College where one of my former classmates teaches. Finding out that I was a nursing educator apparently made her anxious but she didn't say anything to me. Later Dr D said, "She asked me why I didn't tell her!"

Lori did tell me that she knew Janice and that Janice now worked at MGH. I was surprised to hear this. She offered to call Janice and tell her that I was in surgery if I wanted her to. I agreed.

A few minutes later she told me that my former classmate was working and would stop by to see me.

The chief anesthesiologist came into the room. An inexperienced anesthesia resident accompanied him. He explained, "We'll be placing an intravenous line probably in your left hand. Then we'll give you some Versed (a drug that would sedate me). After awhile we'll give you some fentanyl (a drug that would relieve pain)."

He questioned about my experiences with antibiotics because he noted that I was allergic to penicillin and Bactrim. He would give me an antibiotic for surgical prophylaxis (to prevent infection after surgery) later.

He also asked questions about my history with anesthesia. I'd had my tonsils out when I was less than three years old. Apparently other people had horror stories to share. I had none. I had no memories whatever. I even forgot to tell Dr. D that I' had a tonsillectomy as a young child.

As he spoke, he also guided the anesthesia resident through the procedure and advised me that they were now going to give me Versed.

My previous experience with Versed had been amazing. In 1995 I had received Versed prior to having a closed reduction of a fractured foot. It had seemed to me that the actual procedure of fixing the fracture under conscious sedation had taken about two seconds. Although I did not realize it at the time, I had also received fentanyl.

Shortly after I received the Versed, the anesthesiologist said that they'd be giving me fentanyl now. It wouldn't be long before I'd no longer be aware of what was happening.

Suddenly it seemed very crowded in pre-anesthesia room 29. My primary nurse, the anesthesia team, and the surgical resident who would be assisting Dr.

D surrounded me. A woman entered the room shortly after 9:30 AM. I didn't recognize her.

My primary nurse said, "Janice is here." I looked puzzled. Then I realized that she wasn't the Janice that I went to school with. She'd been on the faculty at Boston University when I was a graduate student but I'd never met her.

My last preoperative moments were spent discussing the apparent mix-up and wondering, "Where is that catheter? I've really to go now!" Everything seemed to get quiet. It was shortly after this encounter that I thought that I fell asleep. [In July the anesthesiologist told me, "Oh, you didn't fall asleep in the pre-anesthesia room. We'd not let you until we attached the monitors. It wouldn't be safe."]

At 9:40 AM the anesthesiologists brought me into operating room 29 and gave more medications—cisatracurium and propopol—through the IV tubing. These medications would ease insertion of the tube into my windpipe through which they would give me anesthetic gases and would relax my skeletal muscles so that I wouldn't move about during surgery. I was no longer aware of the events that were taking place. The anesthesiologist also gave me clindamycin (an antibiotic to prevent surgical wound infection). This is standard practice.

After the breathing tube was inserted, they connected it to anesthesia apparatus that enabled them to control the amount of oxygen, nitrous oxide, and forane that I'd need to remain oblivious to the events that were about transpire. Positioning for surgery and a preliminary examination under anesthesia took place. The skin prep was done as close to surgery as possible to minimize the risk of surgical wound infection. A Foley catheter was put in place to insure that the urinary bladder remained empty and tucked away from the surgeons' workspace.

Preparation for surgery was complete. Dr D and her surgical team went to work. Dr D began operating at 10:09 AM and completed the surgery at 12:06 PM. At 12:14 PM I was taken from operating room 29 to the recovery room. For two hours Dr D and her surgical team were very busy. I was not.

After cutting the skin with a knife, they separated fatty tissue and the underlying abdominal muscles using cautery. Cautery is used to seal off tiny blood vessels and to create a bloodless surgical field. The peritoneum looked good. The large left adnexal mass did not. The good news is that the adhesions were loose, the mass was encapsulated, and no enlarged lymph nodes were felt. The surgical team carefully dissected the targeted organs and the mass from surrounding tissue. Care was taken to seal off blood vessels and to protect ligaments, nerves and the tubes that drain the kidneys into the bladder

During oncology surgery a pathologist is present to examine tissue samples. The pathologist confirmed adenocarcinoma. The surgeons proceeded with staging by sampling multiple lymph nodes in the pelvic area and adhesions of the mass to the sigmoid colon (lower bowel) nearby. They also did an appendectomy to eliminate the risk of future rupture resulting in infection and sampled nodes near the aorta—the major artery through which blood is pumped from the heart to the whole body.

As each tissue sample was removed, it was handed off to the circulating nurse who carefully placed it into an individual container labeled with my name and an identifying symbol. Later the pathologists' report would describe the precise status of each distinct specimen. The circulating nurse would also verify with the scrub technician that all instruments and sponges were accounted for before the surgeons closed the wound. This is standard practice. After suturing the underlying muscle and fatty tissue, the surgeons stapled the wound and applied a sterile dressing. The sensations that I experienced while I was in the operating room were strange to say the least. I don't recall seeing anything during this interval but I heard a constant high-pitched droning sound for what seemed to be an undetermined period of time.

The anesthesiologists removed the tube from my windpipe and transferred me to the recovery room at 12:14 PM. A moment later I entered the world of a recovering patient. I was admitted to the Post Anesthesia Recovery Unit.

About 12:25 PM I started to stir. I mumbled, "I can't wait for this catheter any longer. I have to make one last pit stop now!" The recovery unit nurse reassured me, "You are okay. You are in the recovery room. Your operation is over. You have a catheter in place. Relax and try to go back to sleep for awhile. You need to stay here for awhile." She would describe me as disoriented. My sense of time passing had stopped nearly three hours ago. It was as if the train had gone through a very dark tunnel and now I had to adjust to the daylight. When she told me where I was, I knew instantly that I was okay and I settled back.

The nurse may have given me dilaudid (an analgesic) at this time but I'm not sure. From my vantage point in section four I couldn't see much in the recovery room except for the clock on the wall, the pump regulating the intravenous fluid that was flowing into a left arm vein, and the gentle nurse who was monitoring my condition and providing care. A nurse was there. I could relax. I fell asleep.

When I opened my eyes at 2:25 PM the anesthesiologist was reviewing my chart and speaking in a low voice with the recovery room nurse. He looked up and told me, "You're doing very well. You'll be going to your room very shortly." I closed my eyes and fell asleep.

The next flurry of activity that I recall occurred just before 3:00 PM when the nurse told me, "You're still in recovery. We'll be taking you to your room shortly. You did great! Dr D will see you in the morning."

5

Is the Enemy Really Gone?

Shortly after I awoke from anesthesia, two transport aides arrived and took me by stretcher to the nursing unit where I would stay until discharge. During my journey from the recovery room to the nursing unit, I saw very little—the walls and ceilings of the elevator and the long corridors through which we traveled. I remember being awed by the exquisite woodwork in the older buildings. The transport aides were chatting about what they were going to do when they got off duty.

When we arrived at our destination, they asked me, "Can you move onto the bed?"

I said, "No!"

One of them went off to get a transfer team together. When they returned, they went to work and executed the transfer.

Meanwhile, the priest arrived. As the staff prepared to move me into my bed, he asked, "Did you want to talk to me?"

I said, "I was hoping that you would pray with me. A minister saw me and she prayed."

While the transfer team lifted me onto the bed, the priest prayed. The nurse explained how the call bell worked and how the Patient Controlled Analgesia (PCA) Pump worked and then checked my vital signs. For a few minutes it was hectic but it quieted down and I went off to sleep for awhile. I woke up around 4:30 PM and asked to have the telephone so that I could call my mother. I talked a few minutes, told her that I was okay, and said that I'd call her in the morning.

She told me that my brother and his wife were going to come in and visit me that evening.

My brother and his wife arrived around 7:00 PM. I don't remember much about the visit. I recall that they asked if I needed anything. I asked them to bring in something to read—three or four journals from the stack on the dining room table would be fine.

Although a coworker had warned me that the food was bad, I didn't think to ask them for food. That was a big mistake. My brother's wife said, "We're going to bring the kids tomorrow night. We thought that today might be too much." I agreed. They left around 8:00 PM.

I was accustomed to lying on my side and was able to move from side to side easily. One of the nurses commented, "You never seem to be in the same position twice and you look so comfortable." I thought to myself, "I am comfortable. My exercise program really worked out." Although my mobility program was working from my perspective, almost every time I moved, I pulled the call light out of the wall. Several times during the night, the secretary said, "You pulled the call light out of the wall." This was frustrating for the nurses but I was a woman on the move!

Whenever I moved, the compression boots stopped working. I'd adjust my legs so I'd feel the compression boots doing their stuff. preventing a pulmonary embolism (a traveling clot that could block major vessels in the lungs).

The nurse explained how to use the gadget to promote lung expansion. I tried to use it conscientiously. In fact I overused it but I was uncoordinated. Some of the time I wasn't sure that I was using it right. I decided that if I took deep breaths on a regular basis I would expand my lungs sufficiently.

For the most part, my first postoperative night was uneventful. However, I had an episode during which I felt some gushing. It upset me but it was a transient event. The nurse who had been caring for me was going to bring fluids but she forgot. After that the nurse who took over my care didn't give me any more oral fluids during the night. This puzzled me. I wondered, "Do they expect me to bleed again?"

My system for using the PCA pump was unique. As soon as I got comfortable and was ready to try to fall asleep, I pressed the button. I knew that I couldn't overmedicate myself. I didn't want to be awakened by pain. I didn't think that I got much sleep. My sense of time was distorted and I had no idea when I had pressed the PCA button last. I thought that I overheard the nurse say to the resident that she'd given me a bolus—an additional amount of analgesic—because I'd been pressing the button often. No bolus dose was recorded in my medical record.

Around 3:00 AM I saw the nurse doing something to the mini-pump that was hanging by my bed. My perception was that she was starting chemotherapy. Joanna, Dr. D's nurse, had told me that if I needed chemotherapy that I'd receive the first dose in the hospital. I thought to myself, "Oh my God, they are starting the chemotherapy before Dr. D speaks to me. This is wrong. She wouldn't want this. She must've written the orders to have the medication ready to start after she speaks to me. Why did they start this before she told me what's going on? This is absurd. They shouldn't have started it yet."

When the nurse gave me IV Zantac at 9:00 PM, I knew what I had been given. At 3:00 AM, according to my medical record, the nurse had also given me IV Zantac but my imagination of the worst case scenario had taken over.

I changed my position, pulled the call light out from the wall once more, and tried to sleep. I doubted that I slept but I must've slept more than I realized. The amount of medication from the PCA pump that I got on nights was half what I got on evenings. If I were awake during the night, I wouldn't have let that happen.

Shortly after 6:00 AM on January 12th Dr. Henderson the GYN surgical resident arrived. After having minimal conversation with the night nurse, she was a delight. She asked, "How was your night?" She put me at ease. She removed the surgical dressing and I had my first look at the incision. I was almost flat in bed so I couldn't see much. Dr. H told me that Dr. D would arrive shortly and the surgical team that assisted her with my surgery would accompany her. Someone put a chair beside my bed.

About one-half hour later, Dr. D and her surgical team arrived. She asked them to introduce themselves. Even the medical student who didn't have to attend rounds had come in to visit me. I was pleased that she had done so. Meeting the person who had the surgery is so important for students. After discussing my recovery, Dr D suggested that the team move on to the next patient—my roommate.

Dr. D sat in the chair next to my bed and discussed her findings, "You had ovarian cancer."

I was quiet.

She continued, "We got it all. We took out a thousand nodes."

Pointing to my upper outer abdomen, I asked, "Is that why I have pain here?"

She responded, "Yes."

I said, "I wondered why. I don't have any pain around my incision—just here (pointing to the outer abdomen). But I have to wait for the pathology report?"

She spoke again, "Yes. I also took out your appendix." She went on to explain what would happen during my first post-operative day. They would remove the catheter, get me up to the bathroom, and get me walking. She promised "famous Mass General 'jello'". She apparently thought that MGH had a market on awful 'jello'. They definitely don't. Every hospital in the country knows about institutional gelatin. Surviving this gelatin is a rite of passage of the hospitalized.

Not too long after Dr D and her surgical team departed, the nursing staff began to mobilize me. They replaced the chair that Dr. D had used with a more practical chair for a recovering patient and helped me get out of bed for the first time. The nursing assistant brought me a pitcher of water. It was as if I had reached an oasis in the Sahara. I drank a lot of water. My mouth was slow to recover from its stuffed dry cotton effect of having no oral fluids during the night. In spite of the fact that I'd had about five liters or quarts of intravenous fluid in the last 24 hours, my mouth was incredibly dry.

A dietary aide arrived with my breakfast in a timely manner. I was surprised to get what looked like food. I thought, "Wow, I am doing better than I thought! A real breakfast! It was a breakfast tray but the food wasn't real—at least not by most people's definition. The coffee resembled the dredges from a coffee urn that'd been left for a few weeks without being emptied. It could've easily been used to as a seal coat on the temporary road spans for the Big Dig. The cereal that would be promoted as hot was very cold and very tough to chew. It would've made a good Frisbee. The powdered eggs were rubbery and cold as well. The orange juice had been served in a single serve container. It was the only item that was palatable. I thought, "This is really gross but I have to eat if I want to get out of here. I need food if I'm going to get my gut moving!" I ate as much as I could tolerate but it wasn't easy. The developed world would've understood if I'd turned it away.

When the dietary server came to remove my tray, he left a menu. I set survival skills into motion. I ordered two boxes of dry cereal and two cartons of milk, juice, and tea for breakfast. I scrutinized the menu closely for foods that are hard to spoil for lunch and supper and ordered these. I knew that if I were going to escape that I had to eat. The only obstacle to my plan was that I received the house menu for the rest of this day. My choices wouldn't kick in until the next day.

Danika, my nursing assistant, came in and said, "I'm going to bathe you."

"You don't need to. I can do this."

She tried to convince me that I should let her give me a sponge bath. I was adamant that I was going to do this myself. She told me that she wasn't allowed to start another patient until she'd completed her work with me.

Finally she asked hesitantly, "Could I at least wash your back?" I relented and let her do this.

Then Karen, my primary nurse, came in. She had an injection of Lovenox or enoxaparin (a heparin like medication that prevents clot formation) and Colace or docusate (a stool softener). She told me that the catheter would be removed. She said that she could give me an analgesic if I had pain. She could give me a suppository now or later whatever I thought best. At my request she gave me an analgesic at this time and waited until later when I decided that it was time for the suppository.

After she left, I needed to empty my bladder. I decided to go to the bathroom, something that I do not recommend to others. I inadvertently hit the emergency button in the small bathroom with the bulky IV pole. Setting off the emergency alarm always elicits a flurry of activity on a hospital unit, as it should.

I tried to assure the nurses who were running in to check me that I was fine. The first nurse to arrive said, "We have to check for ourselves!" The good news resulting from being able to empty my bladder was that Karen could discontinue the IV. She may have converted the IV catheter to an intermittent lock—a temporary measure that is often taken until the nurses are sure that the patient will tolerate oral fluids.

After Karen discontinued the IV, she said, "I'll ask her if you can have pain medicine by mouth." When she came back, Karen said, "She said that you can take your pain medicine by mouth."

I decided to go back to bed for a little while. When I asked Karen if she had to reattach the pump to the compression boots, she said, "Wait, I'll ask her."

When she returned a minute later, Karen said, "She said that you don't need them anymore."

I was surprised that she returned so quickly. I asked, "Is Dr D still here?"

She laughed, "Oh no, I am checking with Dr. H."

Later Karen came in to take me for a walk. Walking is crucial as it mobilizes the gut and promotes recovery. I was eager to be on my way.

A sightseeing tour through a gynecology unit isn't very exciting. Karen showed me the shower room and said that Dr D would probably let me shower the next day. When she weighed me, I was dismayed to learn that I'd gained ten pounds. She tried to reassure me that this was fluid from surgery and not a permanent weight gain but I was unconvinced. Although I knew that I'd received five liters of fluid and five liters of fluid weighs about ten pounds, I was still dismayed.

Karen told me, "My goal is to have you walk the corridor three times by 7:00 PM."

I said, "Oh, I need to do better than that."

Lunch was an improvement over breakfast. I had chicken, potato, and a vegetable blend—broccoli, carrots, and cauliflower—not the best choice for a postoperative patient. However, all systems were "go."

After lunch I took several walks through the corridor of the gynecology unit and its adjacent corridors. Although I was somewhat adventuresome, I was reluctant to wander too far from my unit, not because I was afraid that my physical ability would interfere with my return but that I wouldn't find my way back. I didn't want the staff to think that I got lost because I was confused. During my journey I discovered that the unit had a family room but it was locked but the family room in the adjacent building was open.

During one of my trips I found Danika and I told her, "I am sorry that I was such a grump this morning." We hugged each other. She was very understanding and forgiving. I wasn't the first grump that she's had to deal with nor would I be the last. The frontline health care workers deal with a lot but they work hard to help us on the road to recovery.

I told Danika, "I found a room in the next building where I can bring the kids this evening so that they won't disturb my roommate." My roommate was very sick. She could meet my family but not be distressed by two exuberant children.

Danika said, "We have a family room on this unit. You have to be buzzed in so that we know where you are and can keep an eye on you." I was delighted to hear this. The family room on our unit seemed to be more kid friendly.

The kids enjoyed their visit. My nephew enjoyed being able to sit back in the lounge chair. My niece thought that being able to make pictures on a special mirror was really cool. Her grandmother didn't understand how she would do this. She said, "Grammy, just watch and learn."

The kids thought that the visit to the hospital was great and liked the gifts that I gave them. I'd brought my own personal care items and didn't need the toothbrush, toothpaste, soap, powder and lotion provided by the hospital.

Karen went home for the night at 7:00 PM and Ali assumed responsibility for my care. She kept a close watch on me and made sure that I didn't have to wait long for pain medication. Once she tucked me into bed for the night I slept like a baby. I barely woke up for vital signs and other assessments.

6

Journeying in Faith

Had it not been for my faith journey I wouldn't have made it through my illness. My faith journey has taken me on a tortuous route. Some aspects of the journey made sense to me. Others didn't. Although my family didn't attend church, I had a longing that goes back to my early childhood. I wanted very much to go to Sunday school.

As a child my parents wanted to surprise me. They were taking me by train to Benson's Wild Animal Farm in New Hampshire, but they told me that they were taking me to Sunday school. Although I had a great time, I was disappointed when I hadn't gone to Sunday school.

Visiting church during my childhood years was a rare event. Patty whose grandmother lived next door asked me to go to church with her whenever she visited her grandmother. My aunt and uncle invited me to vacation at their home every summer. They took me to Mass at St. Ambrose Church. Mass was said in Latin. I didn't understand what was going on. Neither did anyone else. Older women often said the rosary during mass. My uncle's mother, a little Italian woman who had immigrated with her husband several years earlier, lent me rosary beads. I didn't know what to do with them.

Sometimes I stayed overnight with another aunt. She had books that included traditional stories about the life of Jesus as a Child. I found details about His childhood that had been passed down from generation to generation. Later I would learn that none of these stories were included in the Gospels recorded by Matthew, Mark, Luke, and John.

When I was twelve, neighbors who had taken my brother to church with them invited me to their church downtown. I went to that church during my teen and young adult years. As a young adult, I taught Sunday school. For several years Nancy and I conducted the Junior High Youth Fellowship on Sunday afternoons.

Mabel and I coordinated retreats for about 80 young people from the Junior High and Senior High Young Fellowship Groups. Each class of 10–12 young people took turns preparing the meals. Mabel and I grilled hotdogs and hamburgers for the entire group Saturday evening. We surprised the group when we took on this task. We succeeded because we were organized.

Later I took part in the groundbreaking for their new church building when they moved to a residential neighborhood where they could expand their religious education program. I continued to teach Sunday school. Sometimes I assisted in the Nursery or in Junior Church. In those days infants and toddlers were cared for in the Nursery during the entire church service. Sermons could be quite lengthy. Just before the sermon younger children were dismissed and had junior church. Noisy children weren't well tolerated.

A little boy hadn't been taken out of church before the sermon. When the minister mentioned his namesake during the sermon, he jumped up and exclaimed loudly, "How did you know my name? This is the first time I ever came here!" The minister yelled, "Get him out of here!" The little boy had no idea what he had done.

After I graduated from high school I attended a Christian College located in the Fenway area of Boston. Among the subjects that I studied were Old Testament Survey and New Testament Survey. While I attended this college, I worked as a nursing assistant at a nearby teaching hospital. My religious experience played an important part in my life and influenced how I viewed and cared for patients. Other students who were already registered nurses also worked at nearby hospitals. When the college moved their campus to Wenham, I wasn't able to continue to study there.

Later I enrolled in a nursing program in my home town. Prior to entering this program I'd worked as a nursing assistant on the maternity unit. During this time the nurses who worked at this hospital were very aware of the spiritual needs of their patients. The Catholic nurses were very excited when Father Lynch was assigned to be the Catholic chaplain at the Hospital. Under his guidance the

Guild of Saint Catherine for Nurses was founded. Then the Protestant nurses who welcomed Reverend Eldridge to the hospital as Protestant Chaplain were active in starting a local Chapter of the Guild of Saint Barnabas for Nurses. They met monthly at Stephen's Church Episcopal Church. Initially a spirit of competition between the two guilds existed but as time went on, a spirit of camaraderie emerged.

While I was a nursing student we had a group called the Lamplighters. I served as President. I joined the Guild of Saint Barnabas for Nurses and attended the meetings when work or school didn't interfere. My aunt's mother and her aunt both belonged to this Guild. The Guild still meets monthly at Stephen's Church in the afternoon instead of the evening during the spring and fall. I have enjoyed hearing their stories about how nursing was.

After graduation I became a registered nurse. I worked at North Shore Children's Hospital and continued my studies at Boston University School of Nursing. After earning my Bachelor of Science Degree in Nursing in 1966 and a Master of Science Degree in Nursing in 1967, I took a teaching position in a nursing program in Central Massachusetts. Later I taught nursing in the Merrimack Valley region. Doctoral programs in nursing had not been developed and the program chairperson encouraged me to earn a Certificate in Advanced Graduate Studies. I developed a program that met my personal objectives and presented it to the Maternal and Child Health Faculty at Boston University School of Nursing. After they accepted my proposal, I went on to earn a CAGS in 1971.

I taught Nursing of Children for several years in the Tri-City area. My attendance at my hometown church had been sporadic because I no longer lived in the area.

Later while working at Children's Rehabilitation Center, a co-worker invited me to attend a prayer group at the Cenacle Retreat House on Lake Street in Brighton. When my schedule enabled me go to the prayer group, I discovered that she had given me unclear directions and I couldn't find the Cenacle Retreat House.

After passing by the Retreat House several times, I saw a group of people gathering in front of St Ignacius Church near the end of the Green Line across the street from Lake Street. I drove into the parking lot to ask someone how to get where I was going. I discovered that the prayer group was meeting at this church. At this time Pope Paul VI was very ill and a prayer for his recovery was spoken.

The Sisters at the Cenacle Retreat House were on their annual retreat. If I had found the Cenacle Retreat House, they wouldn't have come to the door. I was amazed that I found this group in spite of being unable to find the retreat house.

This prayer group became a very important part of my life for several years. Usually they met at the Cenacle Retreat House. Sometimes they met at St. Clement's Hall at St. John's Seminary. I attended this prayer group regularly until my doctoral studies took me to the University of Rhode Island.

Often priests who were known as healing priests celebrated Mass and prayed with sick members of the prayer community. Although some people appeared to have physical healing, not all did. Most were healed spiritually and derived spiritual strength from their association with the prayer group. I tended to be a cautious skeptic but I would pray with those who desired prayer for healing.

Shortly after my first visit to the Cenacle Prayer Group, I attended a retreat at LaSallette Shrine in Ipswich. During one of the meetings at the retreat I observed that a woman was having periods of breathing difficulty. She'd told me earlier that she had asthma. Several times I prayed quietly for her and her breathing eased. Each time her breathing became more difficult, I prayed and her breathing eased. During the discussion period she told the group, "I've had several healings throughout the afternoon." While I was there, they announced Pope Paul VI died.

I attended another retreat at the Cenacle in the fall. I didn't know anything about the participants. After I arrived, I learned that retreats at the Cenacle are silent. Although I'd met Sister Rita at the prayer group, I got to know her at the retreat. While I was there we found out that John Paul I had died. He had only been Pope for a short while—a month.

In the meantime I'd moved back to the city where I grew up. I went to the local Catholic Church where my mother had gone as a child. I went to the Rectory to enroll as a member of the parish. The secretary told me that Father H would call me. He never did.

I went back a week later. The secretary seemed distraught. The priest whom she said would call me had just died in Europe. He had leukemia. The church was in turmoil. Instead of waiting for another priest to get back to me, I asked Sister Rita, a sister at the Cenacle, to assist me in preparing for the Sacraments. She spoke with Father John G about our plans.

Father Gerard Dorgan who was on the faculty at St John's seminary was the celebrant on November 1st when I received First Holy Communion. He frequently celebrated Mass for the prayer group and provided us with homilies that enlightened us about the Saints and the Sacraments of the church and helped us to grow in faith. When it was announced that the Bishop would be coming to the Cenacle for my confirmation, four other women asked to be confirmed at the same time. A group from the local Catholic Church came to the celebration.

As I continued on my faith journey, I volunteered to teach CCD and taught fifth graders for several years. The children were a diverse group. Some children were from families who took part in the life of the church. Other families that didn't attend church sent children to CCD but not to church. Providing experiences that would meet the spiritual needs of the diverse children who were in this class was challenging.

Mass usually ended fifteen minutes before CCD started. Thus children who came after church would arrive earlier than the children who came from home. I'd ask the children to write or draw what the lesson of the day meant to them. If the lesson was about the Sacrament of Baptism, I would instruct them to "Write or draw something that tells what Baptism means to you."

Most children were able to tell a story describing or draw a picture depicting something to do with Baptism—perhaps the baptism of a little cousin. As soon as everyone had arrived, we could use their stories and pictures as a starting point.

One little boy always drew a picture of something related to the Boston Bruins. Trying to find something in his experience that related to the lessons wasn't easy, but I believed that it was important. I made every effort to make a connection.

Finding ways to help the children discover how much they had learned about the church was important. One way that I did this was by creating a board game called *Journey through Palestine.* The game was designed to help the fifth graders discover how much they'd learned about their faith. The "board" had a map of Palestine and the roads that Jesus traveled during His sojourn on earth. Children could draw cards, depending on where they landed, that addressed different topics that were part of the fifth grade curriculum.

One of the students was puzzled by one of the cards that he drew during the game. It read, "You meet Jesus at the well. Lose one turn." The youngster wanted to know, "Why would you lose a turn if you meet Jesus at the well? Isn't that a good thing?" I used this opportunity to explain that sometimes things in life may seem to be going too fast and we need to slow down, as Jesus did, and let God be present in our life." He seemed to understand.

The Office of Religious Education of the Archdiocese provides a Master Teacher Program in doctrinal and methodological requirements for Religious Education Teachers. Three teachers from our local parish traveled to Newton every Tuesday evening from September to May. When the grade 4–6 coordinator retired, she recommended me for her position. Irma was the grade 1–3 coordinator and Sister B was the grade 7–9 coordinator. We worked as a team. I coordinated these grades until my doctoral studies took me to the University of Rhode Island.

One year we decided to have a Bible Fair as a fundraiser for our community service project. I created a different version of my board game and called it "Crossing the Red Sea." Children could play this game at a fair because it had a shorter time frame. We gave prizes to the children who crossed the Red Sea first.

John C who taught bible study classes in the area played our game at the Bible Fair. He pulled the card that read, "What are the names of the twelve disciples?" If he named all twelve, he could move one space.

Only John would've known to ask, "According to which Gospel? They list different names, you know." We assured him that we'd be flexible. After John's experience, I realized decided that I needed to rank the cards according to level of difficulty for the next time.

I had also become a member of the local prayer group. Several members of this prayer group had cancer and found support in this group.

Occasionally the leaders of the prayer groups would invite healing priests to celebrate Mass and pray for the individual members of the prayer groups. Although I heard stories of physical healing, I only witnessed spiritual healing. Nonetheless I prayed for healing whenever I had an opportunity.

The priests who celebrated Mass for the prayer groups always invited us to include our petitions during the prayers of the faithful. I always prayed for the children at Children's Rehabilitation Center, their families and friends, and the staff who cared for them. Other members of the prayer group would include my petition if I was unable to attend the prayer meeting.

Ordinarily the priests who celebrated daily or Sunday Mass didn't invite parishioners to voice their petitions. In June 1985 while I was attending Mass at the Disabled American Veterans Convention in Springfield, the Bishop who was celebrating Mass invited us to voice our petitions. I accepted his invitation and prayed for the children at Children's Rehabilitation Center, their families, their friends, and the staff who cared for them.

In the meantime the passengers of a TWA flight out of Athens had been taken hostage. While the hostage takers were trying to escort the women and children off the plane, one on the nurses who worked at Children's Rehabilitation Center was refusing to leave her husband who is legally blind behind. Although they were reluctant to release him, they had a change of heart and escorted him off the plane. God worked in a mysterious way to provide an opportunity for the participants in a Mass in Springfield Massachusetts to pray for people in distress half way around the world.

While I was at our hometown prayer group a woman from a neighboring town spoke of her devotion to Blessed Kateri Tekiwatha—a North American Martyr. In the early 1980s I visited the Shrine of the North American Martyrs in Auriesville New York and learned more about her spiritual journey. I enrolled my family at the Shrine and a plaque acknowledging this enrollment is there.

During my darkest moments after learning of my potential diagnoses and possible death, the notion of praying to Blessed Kateri Tekiwatha occurred to me. The likelihood that I needed a major miracle in my life was foremost in my thoughts. The peace of mind that I found was very important to me as I continued on my journey. I remembered the lesson in the game—Journey through Palestine. I had to slow down and let God be present in my life.

During my faith journey God has been present in my life in many ways. God has been present with me, as I have walked through the Valley of Impending Death that initiates the life of Living with a Life Threatening Illness.

As my friends and fellow parishioners learn of my illness, their prayers have filled my life and have offered me encouragement. Although the priest couldn't be there when I entered the surgical unit, a minister was present and prayed intently for my well being. Later the priest arrived and prayed as well.

On Saturday evening after my family left the hospital and I got into bed, I heard my hospital roommate whispering to her adult son who has Down syndrome. He was shy and didn't seem to want to do what she was asking. She persisted.

He approached me and said, "My mother wants me to pray for you. Is it okay?"

I said, "Yes."

The young man was very articulate and touched me by his prayer. Every word was from the heart.

God's attention was constantly being diverted in my direction. Two weeks after my discharge from the hospital, I walked the short distance to my local church.

Barbara looked surprised to see me and asked, "Why are you here? We prayed for you last week because you were so sick?"

I replied, "Why are you amazed? Your prayers have helped."

Our pastor was disappointed to learn that I had cancer and needed chemotherapy.

I said, "You knew that I had cancer."

He said, "I wanted a 100% report."

I replied, "My doctor got everything but the cell is aggressive. This is necessary!"

Three parishioners affirmed their concern for me by giving me a sacramental on Palm Sunday a few months after my surgery. In contrast to Sacraments that are graces that are given by God, a Sacramental is given by the Church to help us in our faith journey.

As I continue on my faith journey, I learn that many more people have included me in their prayers. Each prayer has helped me on the way to recovery.

In turn the opportunity to include others in my prayers is present. An usher in our church had prostate cancer. He is doing well. Another had surgery for stomach cancer. Sadly he had a relapse and died. Recently a woman, the mother of a teen-age girl, had a relapse and died. This is really disheartening.

7

No Place like Home

Shortly after 6:00 AM two days after surgery Dr. H the GYN surgical resident entered my room. I had awakened early. I had no desire to try to go back to sleep. I remembered what the nursing supervisor at my hometown hospital had once said. "When they send us the pink bedspreads, the patients look healthier. When they send us yellow, green or blue, they look jaundiced, or green around the gills, or cyanotic. I wish they'd send pink spreads everyday." My goal was to look healthy when Dr. D. arrived. I put on a pink robe.

Dr. H commented, "You're doing very well. When Dr. D comes in, I am going to recommend a discharge. I can't promise. The team makes the decision."

Nonetheless my spirits were lifted. I sat on the edge of my bed and tried to read a journal but I couldn't focus on reading. This wasn't too surprising. I am not a morning person. The anesthesia and the analgesia were probably still affecting me. I pulled the tray table toward me and took out a deck of cards. I played a game of solitaire.

About a half-hour later Dr. D and her team arrived. She laughed, "When you see your patient sitting up playing solitaire, it's definitely time to send her home." Needless to say I was delighted to cooperate. I couldn't imagine what I'd do for two more days in the hospital.

After breakfast, Karen brought in my discharge papers and reviewed the instructions with me. Dr. H had written prescriptions for pain management and bowel management. I packed my bags and I was ready to roll. My brother came to the hospital as soon as he could. We went by the admitting office to pick up the money that I'd brought with me. The line at the hospital pharmacy was long.

I decided to have my prescriptions filled at the local pharmacy. I was home before noon.

My mother prepared Sunday dinner. It was more than I could eat but it was better than the dinner that I had ordered at the hospital and had happily left behind.

During the next few days my recovery was progressing nicely. Unlike my first night home after breaking my foot in 1995, I had no problem negotiating the stairs. Unlike my preoperative course, I didn't have to make frequent facility visits. I could go 2–4 hours between visits. Although my first meal at home was a bit heavy for me, my appetite returned to normal the next day.

My gut was functioning a little more sluggishly than I would have liked. I had to use the stool softeners and suppositories. I relied primarily on acetaminophen or ibuprofen (non-narcotic pain relievers). Infrequently I took hydromorphone (a narcotic pain reliever).

On Monday night I fell asleep shortly after 11:30 PM and woke up seven hours later. I could hardly walk.

My hip had bothered me on several occasions in the past and the orthopedist who evaluated it had prescribed an injection twice. Today it was worse than it had been then. I used ibuprofen to ease my hip pain. I didn't have abdominal pain.

The following day I had some discomfort in the umbilical region. Although I imagined that it was probably a small bowel obstruction, my bowel regime was effective. That night I had a strange dream. Although I could not remember the details, I woke up mumbling, "those damned Balfours."

"Balfours" are heavy metal of the worst kind. Balfours are retractors that protect some tissue from the surgeon's tools and keep it from interfering with surgery. Later I learned that "Balfours" were not used. A Bookwalter retractor was used for this purpose. I felt better thinking that I had a reasonable explanation for my discomfort.

The high-speed express train seemed to be slowing down or so I thought.

The telephone rang shortly after lunch on January 17th. It was Dr. D. Her voice didn't convey the sound of relief. She spoke softly but clearly, "This is Dr. D. I have the results of the pathology report. You have a clear cell carcinoma, grade three. This is an aggressive cell. You need to have chemotherapy."

I couldn't say anything at first. The high-speed express train had suddenly accelerated at an incredible speed.

She continued, "Do you understand what I am saying?

When I was able to respond, I said, "Yes." I couldn't say much.

She asked, "Are you okay with this?"

Although I said, "Yes", I am sure that she knew that I was not okay.

I asked, "Can this be done at North Shore?"

She hesitated, then spoke, "There are some protocols that they can't do there. I can refer you to a medical oncologist if you want."

I said, "Okay." I didn't think that I'd be able to get intown very easily for the chemotherapy. This seemed to be a better alternative for me. I was quiet.

She asked, "Is something else on your mind?"

I hesitated. Then I said, "No, I knew it. I knew that I'd be diagnosed with some type of cancer. It seemed inevitable. I just didn't expect this."

Dr D said softly, "You thought that it might be endometrial cancer?"

"Yeah, I think so, I don't know." After another silence, I said, "These staples are driving me crazy. I don't think that I can stand them until Tuesday. I thought that I would be able to."

She said, "You don't need to wait. Come in tomorrow. I'll have Joanna talk with you so that you can arrange a time."

When Joanna came on the line, she told me, "Come in anytime that you can get a ride. Just call me in the morning and let me know what time so that I'll be here. I don't want you to wait while I'm on break."

The following day was a warm day—very warm for January. No one was wearing heavy winter jackets. Not even me. My brother drove me into Boston. He left me at the entrance and went to park his van. I went in and followed the signs to the Cox building. As I walked through one building to the next, I was amazed by the hustle and bustle of the MGH complex. I saw Mary Lou. I know her from Children's Rehab. She is in charge of the Children's Hospital within a Hospital. They are celebrating its accomplishments with a cake that'll be cut later. We are excited to see each other. When she learns about my recent surgery, she wants to know why I didn't tell her that I was coming in. She tells me that she works closely with the nurses on Bigelow 7. It was good to see her. I continued on my journey to the Cox Building and took the elevator to the fifth floor.

After checking in, an assistant directed me to an examining room and checked my vital signs. Joanna removed the staples. Some staples weren't easy to remove. She thought that the wound was infected.

When the wound was opened, very pale yellow drainage poured forth. Joanna asked the nurse practitioner to look at the wound. The nurse practitioner thought that it was a fat necrosis. Although I didn't know at that time what a fat necrosis was, I didn't think that the wound was infected.

Joanna told me, "The VNA will need to come in to do your dressings. Do you have a preference? I'll give you supplies to hold you over until they come in."

I suggested, "NSVNA. They're affiliated with NSMC."

Meanwhile Dr D was in the operating room. The nurse practitioner suggested that Joanna try to contact her to have her look at it between cases.

When Dr. D saw the incision, she agreed that it should heal by secondary incision (from the inside out) but she wanted to put in a few supporting sutures. While she waited for Joanna to obtain an instrument, she asked me, "How did you come to the hospital?"

I replied, "My brother brought me."

As she worked, she told Joanna to schedule me for "rechecks" to insure sufficient wound healing before chemotherapy.

While I was making an appointment for a recheck, my brother was standing in the hallway. On her way back to the operating room, Dr. D stopped to talk with him. My brother was impressed that she took the time to meet him. He was amazed at her youthful appearance.

Over the weekend, abundant, copious, profuse drainage saturated the dressings. At first I couldn't manage to change the inner packing so I removed and replaced the outer dressings.

The nurse who came on Saturday replenished my supplies and put in an order to a supplier. They were supposed to deliver supplies. The supplies never came.

On Monday the nurse who came was a wound specialist. She wasn't been assigned to me. She was helping a colleague who had a heavier load. We recognized each other. She'd been a preceptor for one of my nursing students. I was relieved to see her. She'd know if my wound was okay.

She put duoderm on my skin so that the nurses could tape the dressings to it instead of to my skin. This spared me the agony of having tape pulled off every day and preserved skin integrity.

She told me, "I know Dr. D. I've worked with her. Dr D made a diagnosis on someone whom I know when no one else could." She told me what I already knew. She is very good at what she does!

I told her that I had a mirror that I could use to try to do dressing changes. She suggested that I try to change the dressing. She'd evaluate how I managed. I tried to change the dressing while I was lying down. I failed miserably.

Later that day I had a brainstorm. I tried to change the dressing while standing. At first I lost a few gauze pads but I learned how to change the packing and the outer dressings. When I was on the other side of the looking glass, the dressing procedure was the reverse of what I was familiar with.

The following day I began to have fever spikes. This wasn't good. I spoke with the resident on call. I'd met him in pre-anesthesia room 29 before surgery and in my hospital room after surgery. He said. "If the fevers continue, come into the emergency room." A trip to the ER in the middle of the night was definitely not on my wish list.

I was circling in a holding pattern waiting for the precise moment when I could take the next step. Meanwhile my first visit with Dr. S was January 22nd. Moving forward with chemotherapy had been tucked in between my visits to my GYN oncology surgeon and her staff. I was trying hard not to crossover but I wasn't able to stop myself. I was on the other side of the looking glass and I didn't like it. I wanted to go back to being a nurse.

I felt at ease with Dr. S. After he asked me a lot of questions, he began the physical examination. He really probed deeply when he examined my underarms and my groin. I knew that if any bad nodes were hiding out he would discover them. On the other hand he was very gentle when he examined my abdomen, taking caution not to cause discomfort where I had my surgery.

He explained that Ricky the nurse practitioner would contact me to arrange the teaching that precedes chemotherapy. They would see me on alternate visits and collaborate in the management of my care.

I'd thought that Dr. D would still be at NSCC but she had left early. Dr. S warned me not to ignore fever if it returned.

My temperature spiked again on the 23rd. I called Joanna and she told me to come in as soon as I could. The weather was still unseasonably warm and people were still dressing very lightly. I decided to wear a sweater and a winter coat. My brother was still available and he drove me to MGH for another assessment.

The volume of drainage was subsiding. The drainage was still very pale yellow. It was now very scant. Joanna swabbed the wound for a culture (to see if any bacteria were present) and obtained a prescription for levoquin (an antibiotic, in case any bacteria were present). This is standard practice.

While my brother went to get his van, I waited near the garage entrance. The day was so nice that everyone was running about in scrubs or white coats. I was dressed for a frigid winter day. I was so cold that I was shivering. My body was shaking. It felt like an earthquake. The heat in the van helped a little. I had the prescription filled on the way home and I started the antibiotic immediately.

After I arrived home, Ricky called and arranged for me to see her the next day for teaching.

I was compelled to confront the fever spikes aggressively. The minute I started to feel slightly cool, I bundled myself. My mother lent me a very heavy sweater—one that would ordinarily be too heavy to wear inside. I wrapped myself in the sweater and covered myself with heavy quilts. If I could prevent the chills, I could halt the fever invasion. My approach to the fever spikes was effective. No more fevers. I won the battle against the fevers. I kept up this nightly ritual for the next week!

Ricky greeted me in the waiting area the next day and suggested that we go upstairs. She led me into a large conference room. Inside the room were a large oval conference table and a dozen comfortable conference chairs.

Ricky offered me a seat at a smaller round table just inside the door. She had my medical record and a stack of papers. I knew that this was serious business.

She explained everything that you'd ever want to know about chemotherapy. She began by showing me a form on which Dr S had written his goal for me and emphasized, "Notice that he has written as the goal for you "CURE!" The letters were one inch tall!

As I had anticipated, I would be receiving paclitaxel (Taxol) and carboplatin (Paraplatin). I would come to the Cancer Center on the designated day and receive these drugs over a 5–6 hour period. I would receive these drugs every three weeks for a total of six times. These medications have a number of potential side effects.

Ricky explained that I needed to come to the Cancer Center 48 hours before I received chemotherapy for standard laboratory work and an assessment. I would be monitored closely and dosages would be calculated on the basis of my weight at this time, changes in blood cell counts and other tests included in the oncology panel, and any physical findings.

In addition, I'd be given medications to minimize some of the more worrisome side effects of the medications. I would take dexamethasone (an anti-inflammatory drug) the evening before and the morning of my chemotherapy. In addition to the antineoplastic (anticancer) medications, I would be receiving other medications (diphenhydramine, lorazepam, cimetidine, and ondansetron) during each day at the cancer center. After each chemotherapy day I would take ondansetron at 8 PM and 8 AM for a total of seven doses by mouth to prevent the onset of nausea. In addition to being given prescriptions for dexamethasone and ondansetron that I took as directed, I was given prescriptions for lorazepam and prochlorperazine that I took as needed to alleviate nausea. Ondansetron effectively prevents nausea and vomiting in most people. I didn't use either lorazepam or prochlorperazine.

The drugs that I received with my chemotherapy, as Ricky explained it, would ward off serious side effects or adverse effects as the medical world describes them. These included heart effects and allergic reactions. The Cancer Center was fully prepared to deal with these effects if they did occur. For me they never did.

When I visited Dr. D for the first time, I'd seen the strategically located crash cart. As a nurse I always surveyed health care settings so that I would be able to respond in an emergency. The fact that I wasn't there as a nurse didn't matter. As a nurse I needed to know where the critical equipment was. I couldn't look at the Cancer Center from the other side of the looking glass.

Today was different. Not only was the high-speed express traveling at an accelerated speed, it was taking me further and further behind the looking glass. Ricky seemed to sense this as she stopped from time to time and looked away. She shuffled through the papers as if to remind herself of what she needed to say. Yet, she seemed to know everything that needed to be included.

Ricky told me about several additional side effects that unlike those mentioned earlier were for the most part relatively inconvenient annoyances. She suggested simple measures to deal with these annoyances.

People on chemotherapy sometimes get sores in their mouth. Hard candy helps. Some people have complained of a metallic taste. Using plastic utensils may be helpful. Joint and muscle pain is possible. Glutamine 10 mg three times a day for four days after chemotherapy may be helpful. Numbness and tingling of the hands and feet may occur. Vitamin B6 50 mg three times a day may help.

She reviewed the information on five pre-printed cards that are given to all patients who seek services at the Cancer Center. The topics include Nutritional Information, Loss of Appetite, Mouth and Throat Pain, Nausea and Vomiting, and GI Problems (heartburn, diarrhea, and constipation). Much of this information is included in Everyone's Guide to Cancer Therapy: How Cancer is Diagnosed, Treated, and Managed Day to Day.

Ricky also reviewed the problems that accompany bone marrow suppression. During chemotherapy the bone marrow goes on vacation and fails to produce sufficient red blood cells, white blood cells, and platelets to meet our health requirements. Fatigue results from insufficient red blood cells or anemia. Lack of protection against infection is a consequence of inadequate white blood cells or leucopenia. Bleeding results from platelet deficiency or thrombocytopenia. She reminded me that the one of blood samples was a complete blood count and it was to determine how well my blood cells were holding out during chemotherapy.

For the most part Ricky talked about possibilities—side effects or adverse effects that **might** happen. Then, not unexpectedly, she said, "You **will** lose your hair." This sounded like an actuality not a possibility and this comment was distressing.

Of course, I knew that alopecia (hair loss) was an expected side effect of chemotherapy. I had also seen the media publicize how the local kids rallied around their sick friend who lost all of his or her hair and had their hair shaved as well. I had seen women wearing their turbans or wigs.

As Ricky explained about hair loss and the cranial prosthesis (the mysterious name that the third party payers give to wigs), I thought passionately, "I will not lose my hair." Ricky said, "It usually starts to fall out in about 2–3 weeks. Women find it easier if they get their hair cut short before it starts to fall out."

Before I left, I told Ricky that if I were cleared the following Thursday for chemotherapy, I would be able to start on February 14th. She made a note of this in my medical record.

Ricky said, "We have one more thing to do before you leave today. One of the nurses will check your arm to see if you have some good sites for chemotherapy. If you do, you will not need to have a port." A port is a device that is implanted under the skin; it provides for access into the vein where the medication is administered.

Michelle examined the veins in my left arm and wasn't satisfied with the veins on this arm. She said, "Let me look at your other arm." While she was checking my right arm I told Ricky and Michelle that in the past I didn't let anyone use my right arm.

After donating blood I had a large bruise. The nurse at the donor center who'd tried to insert the catheter had trouble finding the vein and had to search for it. As a result the hole in the vein wasn't under the hole in the skin. Usually this doesn't happen. The nurse who removed the catheter wasn't aware of the other nurse's search for the elusive vein. She applied the pressure dressing over the hole in the skin rather than over the vein. Bleeding under the pressure dressing resulted in a painful arm for days.

After that I told the blood donor center nurses, "Either take it from my left arm or not at all. I am saving my right arm for emergencies only." As Michelle counted out six possible sites for inserting a catheter, she said, I think she'll be okay for IVs. I commented, "I think that this is the emergency for which I was saving my right arm."

Ricky said, "Everything's done now. As soon as you are cleared, I will set up your appointment and have you come in for your blood work. We calculate your medications on the basis of your weight and blood work."

As we walked back to the waiting area, Ricky said, "I know, it's overwhelming. This is my card. If you have any questions or concerns, please call me."

My sister-in-law and my great-niece were waiting for me. My great-niece was acquainting herself with the tropical fish in the aquarium. Whenever she or her brother came to the cancer center, they would spend time checking on the status of the fish—which ones were still there, which ones were missing, which ones were new.

Joanna checked my wound on January 25th. She wanted Dr. D to look at it before she removed the sutures. When she entered the examination room, I saw a big difference between the last time I saw her and today. She looked tired and lacked her usual energy. I thought, "Wow, that kid's almost here." After she checked me, I said, "I want to wish you the best of luck with your baby and thank you for everything."

She commented, "Oh, I'll probably see you next week. Come in Wednesday."

I remarked, "Oh, you're going to have that baby Tuesday!" I wasn't that certain that she would wait until Tuesday. I wanted her to have the baby on my niece's birthday so I'd remember the date. I was still confused about the dates. My niece's birthday was twelve days away rather than five days away.

Joanna wanted me to make an appointment for the next Thursday so that a physician would be available. Instead of making an appointment for the 31^{st,} I made it for the following week.

Dr. D's baby made his grand entry in the late evening on January 28th. I was happy to hear that both were doing well.

In the meantime Ricky had seen through my confusion and called to tell me that I would be ready to start chemotherapy a week sooner than I'd said. However, it didn't occur to me that I'd made an appointment with Joanna on the wrong date.

When I came in to see Joanna on January 31st, the receptionist said that I didn't have an appointment. After making a call, she told me to wait. While I waited, I observed other women coming and going. On earlier occasions I wondered, "What kind of cancer does she have? What stage is she in?" Now I wondered, "What kind of treatment is she having? How is she managing with the treatment and its effects?" I was particularly interested in how the women managed hair loss.

Most women were stylishly dressed and appeared as if they were passing by in the middle of their workday. I never saw any women with wigs. I saw some women who had designed their own hair coverings. They had wrapped gorgeous silk pieces casually around their heads and it was hard to tell whether they did or didn't have hair. Watching them was like watching a fashion parade. If I'd seen them elsewhere, I wouldn't even have given them a second thought.

A few women looked ill and didn't appear to be able to continue all of their usual activities. For the most part people weren't kept waiting for long and I didn't see a lot of women on any given day.

Joanna was able to see me when she returned from break. My wound was healed. Chemotherapy was a go! Now I'm really scared.

8

Heroes in the Face of Adversity

The high-speed express train had slowed down but I wasn't able to disembark. Visions of heroes from my past interrupted me as I think about what awaited me. Some of my heroes are the courageous children whom I've known throughout my career as a maternity and children's nurse. Josh is one of those heroes. He recruited me to be his special nurse and I could never forget him.

When I graduated from nursing school, I went to work in North Shore Children's Hospital (NSCH) where I met Josh. NSCH had its origins on nearby Baker's Island in 1904 and was known as the Babies Summer Hospital. Later it expanded to become a year round hospital near Ropes Point. As the mission of the hospital changed and improved standards of care mandated additional resources, the hospital moved to its new location adjacent to the larger local hospital not long before I arrived in September 1963. In 1963 I could work in the role of graduate nurse until I took the State Board Examinations and became licensed as a registered nurse.

The Director of Nursing was responsible for my orientation to the hospital. She was telling me about its history when a nursing instructor interrupted us to tell her that Josh was holding her student at bay. I envisioned a six-foot tall, 200 pound adolescent resisting the efforts of a nursing student to care for him.

When the Director of Nursing introduced me to Josh, I met a tiny child who weighed about 30 pounds and was about 2 ½ feet long. He was in hospital pajamas and was lying in bed. He wore a cowboy hat. An iron lung was next to his bed. He didn't display any interest in meeting me. This would change.

The following week I began my job as charge nurse on the third floor at NSCH. In fall 1963 staffing was excellent. Although I was the designated charge nurse, a registered nurse was always assigned to the unit. Several practical nurses worked on the unit. Not counting the charge nurse, the staff-patient ratio was 1:4.

Josh had his favorite nurses. One of the four practical nurses that he'd allow near him was always scheduled to work. Josh had good reason to be leery of new staff. He had cervical spine instability. On two separate occasions while his dad was carrying him his loosely connected neck bones slipped over one another and pinched off his spinal cord. He developed partial paralysis. Josh wouldn't let everyone touch him. Only those whom he trusted could get near him.

In the meantime Josh and I developed a close relationship. One evening he asked me to draw a picture of an airplane and tape it to his mirror. Prior to this evening my artistic pursuits were limited to "trees" and "cathedrals" or things that I learned to draw in the seventh grade. I wasn't an artist. The night was busy and I didn't have much time to meet this request. However, I found myself waiting on the telephone for the physician whom I had called to come to the telephone. I started to draw an airplane. It turned out well. Josh was delighted. He asked me to tape it to his mirror where it remained while he was at the hospital.

In spite of his immobility Josh had a lot of friends. One of his best friends was "Jack, the Mailman". A nurse who worked on the third floor had a husband who was a mailman. He used to talk to her about a little boy on his route. Pat used to talk lovingly to him about a little boy on the third floor. One day they realized that they were both talking about Josh.

Several weeks after I met Josh, none of his four special nurses were working. Another practical nurse was assigned to care for him. He knew her and allowed her to take care of him. She came to me at 7:45 PM and said, "It's time for Josh to go into the iron lung and I have never done it before."

As we walked to his room, I thought to myself, "Neither have I! Am I going to be able to do this? What if he won't let me lift him? What will I do? I had no idea!"

When I entered the room I asked, "What time is it?"

Josh answered, "Time to go in!"

I asked, "And how are you going to get in?"

He smiled and pointed to me and said, "You!"

Josh developed a close relationship with me. Now he trusted me. I lifted him and placed him gently into his iron lung.

Within the next few months Josh's mother had to make a very important decision. She could do nothing and let him spend the rest of his days in bed and the rest of his nights in an iron lung. Or, she could consent to surgery that would stabilize the loosely connected bones in his neck. This would prevent the bones from sliding over one another and pinching off his spinal cord again.

After considering the options she said, "I know my son. He would be upset if he grew up and learned that I didn't allow the surgery that might enable him to be mobile." She believed that she was doing the right thing and she knew that the surgery was accompanied by risks.

Josh was transferred to Children's Hospital where he would have spinal surgery. I visited him often.

Before he had his surgery, he'd been placed in a room where he had a great view of the corridor. I was chatting with him. Suddenly he asked me, "What are they going to do?"

I looked up and saw the medical team that was making rounds. They did have a foreboding look about them as they lingered in the hallway several doors down and whispered among themselves. Josh had taught me what the cluster of well-meaning physicians and nurses looked like from the other side of the looking glass.

Before he had his surgery Josh developed pneumonia. They isolated him in a private room in another area of the hospital complex. When I located him, he was in a small room with bare green walls. He was lying between white sheets in a white hospital crib. The room didn't resemble the cheerful surroundings at NSCH. He looked at me and at the walls. He said, "Let's decorate!"

In anticipation of his request, I had red construction paper, white doilies, scissors, and tape. As I cut out hearts, he chose where to tape them. I didn't get the sense that the staff appreciated my efforts as much as Josh did, but I didn't care. A child's room should look as if a child lived there!

During his postoperative recovery, Josh was in Halo traction. He required "one: one" nursing care. Usually either Ms E or Ms F was assigned to Josh. I noticed that Ms. E told Josh what she was going to do and was very gentle with Josh but Ms. F never spoke to him and was abrupt with him. Whenever Ms. E was taking care of him, he called me by name but whenever Ms. F was assigned to him he called me nurse.

One day when he called me nurse, Ms. F spoke curtly to him, "I'll do it when I'm ready." Josh said, "I'm not talking to you. I'm talking to Ms. Downey. You're no nurse."

This little five-year-old validated what I already knew. Telling the child what you are going to do and being gentle with him or her is what nursing is about.

Josh developed pneumonia again. Treatment via an intermittent positive pressure breathing (IPPB) machine had been prescribed. Unfortunately Josh had a problem with his lungs and his lungs didn't withstand the pressure of the IPPB machine. I was upset to learn that my little friend had died.

Tom is another one of my heroes. Unintentionally Tom seemed to follow me wherever I went for several years. By showing courage in the face of adversity, Tom was able to overcome a severe head injury and regain his childhood.

Tom is a 14-year-old who was riding a mini-bike in a schoolyard near his home near the Concord River when he crashed. He was brought by ambulance to the emergency room of a hospital nearby. He was unconscious and unstable. He had a fractured femur. After stabilization in the emergency room and a week in the intensive care unit, he was transferred to the adolescent unit. He was being fed formula through a tube that went through his right nostril into his stomach. His right leg was in traction to stabilize the broken thighbone until it healed sufficiently to allow casting. His room was directly across the hall from my office. I had a good view to monitor his progress.

Tom didn't awaken from coma. Both parents had been divorced and were remarried. His mother was angry and blamed his father who'd let him ride the mini-bike for her son's injuries. The family worked together to facilitate Tom's rehabilitation.

Tom was referred to Children's Rehabilitation Center where he emerged from coma and make considerable progress toward recovery. Both parents and stepparents were involved with his care at the center where Tom made considerable progress.

Sadly Tom's mother who'd had primary custody of her son yielded custody of her son to his father so that he would be eligible for rehabilitation in this state.

Tom was transferred to a pediatric nursing home in his hometown for further rehabilitation and attended the local school daily. He was able to go home to his father's home regularly. He saw his mother who lived out of state less frequently.

I used to see Tom at carnivals and other events that were held for children with disabilities in his hometown. I haven't seen him for several years now.

Kyle, an adorable five-year-old who had a brain tumor, is also a hero. After recovery from surgery Kyle was transferred to Children's Rehabilitation Center. He had multiple problems. He was dependent on oxygen through a tracheostomy (breathing tube), nutritional supplements through a gastrostomy (feeding tube), was prone to seizures, wore braces and was wheelchair dependent. No matter what happened, Kyle would get back on track and continue on with life.

During the night Kyle received chest physiotherapy and inhalation therapy to keep his air passages open and supplemental feedings and anti-seizure medications though his feeding tube to promote growth and prevent seizures. During the day Kyle tool part in a variety of activities—occupational therapy, physical therapy, recreational therapy, respiratory therapy, and speech and language therapy. I rarely thought of Kyle as a child with cancer. My nursing activities were focused on the aftermath of his cancer, its surgery, and its impact on his life.

Most nights were relatively uneventful. Occasionally Kyle would have an episode that required emergency nursing intervention but Kyle would bounce back quickly. What a kid! One of my fondest memories of Kyle took place after an episode at about 6:30 AM. The time involved in stabilizing Kyle resulted in my being unable to complete my other nursing activities on time and being later than usual leaving for the night.

As I left the unit, I saw Kyle wheeling himself into the elevator as he headed for recreational therapy. He waved cheerfully and called out, "See you tonight." I lost a few hours sleep and was tired when I came to work the next night while Kyle had a great day and a great night.

Prior to my arrival several weeks later Kyle had a life-threatening episode. His condition had deteriorated rapidly and the transport team was working to stabilize him prior to his transfer to the referring hospital.

Although the transport team was responsible for his care during transit, the nursing supervisor assigned me to accompany him. Often Kyle would hold his breath during life-threatening episodes. Usually children who hold their breath will breathe again. However, Kyle's protective mechanisms were compromised as a result of his surgery and his breath holding behavior often put him in jeopardy. Tonight was no exception. As the ambulance made its way to children's hospital, Kyle held his breath. The transport physician tried to entice Kyle to breathe but he wouldn't breathe.

I spoke firmly, "Kyle, at the count of three, breathe. Or you will be doing chair time instead of going to 'rec'! One, two..." "Good boy," exclaimed one of the team members.

The transport physician was amazed! After we settled Kyle in his room, she said, "You should see the work that this woman does at the Children's Rehab. I was in awe of the work that the transport team and the staff at the children's hospital were doing. I could never do what they were doing. Yet the physician was praising the work that we did.

Kyle and other children who had been referred to Children's Rehabilitation Center from various tertiary hospitals in the northeast were living with the sequelae of brain cancer. They were some of my heroes.

Other children and adolescents who had traumatic brain injury and had been referred to Children's Rehabilitation Center from diverse tertiary hospitals in the northeast were also some of my heroes.

Sara L was a 17-year-old who had been a passenger in a motor vehicle accident. She had a traumatic brain injury and was comatose. She was an attractive young woman with thick long reddish brown hair that had been braided when she was transferred to Children's Rehabilitation Center. Soon after her arrival I learned at report that a nursing student had shampooed her hair and wasn't able to comb it out. Her hair was incredibly matted. We wondered if we would be able to comb it out without having to cut her hair.

Usually I took care of Sara and her roommate every night. I would not be able to on this night because other children who were on the unit needed my care. When I came to work the next night, I learned that Patti, the evening supervisor, had spent every spare minute she had that evening combing out Sara's hair. Patti did a great job and Sara looked beautiful.

Sara had showed signs of lightening (indications that she would be waking up from her coma) for some time but she wasn't waking up as we'd expected. I was baffled. I kept saying, "I thought that she would wake up!" Jan agreed.

One night I was in Sara's room and someone called me from the nurses' station. I said, "Wait a minute!" This person called me again and again. I repeated somewhat crossly, "I'll be there in a minute!" As I turned, I saw Sara's expression. She looked startled. I couldn't believe it. Then, as quickly as her expression appeared, it disappeared. She appeared as expressionless as she'd been since her admission.

I started babbling to her, "Sara, I didn't mean to frighten you. I was talking to someone else. Don't be afraid! Sara, you are in the hospital. You had an accident. I think that you're awake but you're afraid because you don't know where you are. You need to start talking to us so we can help you to get well." Sara didn't answer.

I thought that I might have imagined it. After all I had wanted her to wake up so badly. I didn't say anything about my observations to anyone.

When I came to work the next night, Jan came running into the nurses' station to give me report. She was a few minutes late. The first words out of her mouth were, "Guess who started talking today."

"Sara L." I responded.

"How'd you know?" Jan queried.

I told her about the encounter that I'd had the night before. I said, "I didn't want to say anything because I wasn't sure if I imagined it or not."

Jan laughed, "Well, you didn't imagine it. She's been talking a blue streak. We haven't been able to stop her."

Not all children and adolescents with traumatic brain injury wake up from their coma. Seventeen-year-old Bud and sixteen-year-old Marie were among those who never woke up. Their mothers came in every day to see them. Usually I saw them on Saturday, as I was the nursing supervisor on Saturday. Saturdays were usually quiet because most of the children went home on Saturday morning and returned Sunday evening. One Saturday as I entered the unit I was about twenty feet behind them as the women were returning to the unit after lunch.

I couldn't hear most of their conversation but I heard Marie's mother say to Bud's mother, "No one knows what a mother goes through!" Bud's mother nodded, "I know." Their mothers are "heroes in the face of adversity". They spend time with their children talking to them and caring for them. Their children do not awaken.

Not all of my heroes at Children's Rehabilitation Center had serious physical illnesses or traumatic injuries. Children in the cognitive behavioral inpatient program had behavioral, interactional, and learning difficulties. Five-year-old Zachary came from a dysfunctional family and wasn't able to go home on the weekends. Usually one of the counselors took him out for the day on Saturday and again on Sunday. Going to a house was important and his mother gave permission to the staff so that he could visit their homes on the weekend. I had the opportunity to take him for the day on a Saturday. I asked him what he wanted to do. He wanted to go on a picnic and he wanted to visit my tall house.

We packed a picnic lunch and went to the Stone Zoo where we visited the animals and had our picnic lunch. Visiting the Stone Zoo was a great experience for Zachary because he could see everything in a relatively short time period. Then he could enjoy our picnic before we headed out to my tall house. On the way we would stop at Toys R Us to get his reward and the local supermarket to buy food for our supper.

Zachary had worked very hard during the week and had earned a reward. He wanted an airplane. When he went to the Kids' Store to get his reward, there were no airplanes left. He didn't want anything else.

We saw two small airplanes at Toys R Us. I tried to steer him toward the better-made one of the two but he was adamant that he wanted the other. We bought the one that he chose.

Then we went to the local supermarket to buy food for supper. He wanted to make pancakes and pour lots of syrup on the pancakes. He also wanted to make strawberry short cake.

Zachary was surprised to discover toys at my tall house because he knew that I didn't have children. I told him that my nieces and nephews played with them whenever they visited. He spent hours playing with a small dump truck under our dining room table. He borrowed a small sugar dispenser to pretend to pour sand in his dump truck and transport the sand to his construction site. Zachary kept me informed about his progress as he went about his activities.

When suppertime came, we made pancakes and poured lots of syrup on them. He'd helped me prepare the strawberries earlier so that they'd be sweet when we're ready to make the strawberry shortcake. He explained that he knew what to do because he had learned to do these things in cooking. He made great strawberry shortcake.

After supper, I told him how much time we had before we had to drive back to the Children's Rehabilitation Center. Zachary asked me to read some stories to him. During the ride back, he was playing with his airplane. It didn't work the way that he thought it would. He was disappointed. He said, "I should've taken the one that you told me about."

I told him that even if the airplane didn't work the way that he thought it would, he could power it himself. He could use his imagination the same way he did when he played with the dump truck. It wasn't his fault that the advertising was misleading.

It was important that I let Zachary know that he had earned the airplane by doing a great job all week. He earned the right to choose and his choice was important. We tried to think of places where he could imagine flying his airplane.

It was time to get ready for bed when we returned to Children's Rehabilitation Center. He asked the staff if I could stay and read a story if he got ready for bed quickly. After reading him a story, I said good night to my little hero and went home to my tall house.

After his sojourn in the CBIP Zachary moved on to another setting. From time to time the staff would update me about the progress that other children who'd been in the program were making in their current schools. I never heard anything about how Zachary was doing.

The head nurse told me this story about another little boy who had been the program. Hyperactivity was one of his problems. He'd been eligible for adoption but no placement had been forthcoming. After his stay in the program, he was placed with a foster family in Southeastern Massachusetts. The principal in his new school had been trying to adopt. This little boy captured his heart and he adopted him. He fit into this family and thrived in his new home. He was transformed from being hyperactive to being more typically active for a child his age.

A grandmother was raising still another little boy in the program. We ran into each other when she had come to take Nick home for the weekend. We knew each other because we belong to the same organization. I met her on the unit when she came to take him home for the weekend. She was happy to learn that she knew someone who worked at Children's Rehabilitation Center.

Nick had made great progress while he was in the program and returned to his grandmother's home. Whenever we attend meetings and conventions, she eagerly seeks me out and provides me with updates on his progress. She was bursting with pride when she told me that he made the honor roll in high school. She couldn't contain her exuberance when she told me that he had graduated from college.

Knowing that even one young man who needed the intense interdisciplinary approach of this unique program has done so well is affirming. I hope to hear more of these stories.

On a more personal level, hearing stories about how people who've had cancer do is also affirming. As I struggled initially with the potential diagnosis of cancer, I wondered, "Does everyone have cancer?" It seemed as if every day I was hearing about someone else who had cancer. After a long struggle with breast cancer, a classmate from nursing school had died from breast cancer. Another classmate died a few years later from a beta cell lymphoma. I didn't even know that this form of lymphoma existed. A third classmate died of lung cancer last year. A fourth one died at the City of Hope in Duarte California. None of my classmates are living with cancer. Only me!

My cumulative life experiences with cancer had convinced me that an early death was an inevitable consequence. I had to learn that life after cancer was a real possibility.

9

Living in Spite of Cancer

My past experiences as a practicing nurse and a nurse educator and as an active member of professional nursing and health organizations served as a backdrop for my journey while I was traveling on the high speed express train. While my cancer was growing silently, turmoil was erupting in one of the nursing organizations in which I'd been active for several years. My sojourn as president of one of its districts would have come to an end at about the time that my cancer was beginning to make its presence known.

Becoming president of the district wasn't part of my plan when I was recruited initially. In spring 1997 Roxanne had called me. As long as I could remember, Roxanne had been the backbone of the nominating committee of our District in the State Nurses Association.

Roxanne promptly revealed the purpose of her call, "We are seeking a candidate for President of the Board of Directors of the District. You've been second vice president. You know the District. Would you consent to serve?"

I knew that it was difficult to recruit qualified candidates because nurses had always had such busy and unpredictable schedules. Their work schedules were getting worse by the day. After serving two terms as second vice president of the Board of Directors, I'd stepped down as required by the By-laws. I could've chosen to run for an office this year but I wasn't thinking of running just yet. I hesitated.

Roxanne continued, "With all the changes at the state level we need someone who's already served on the Board, someone who knows the district. You've been on the Board and you know the State…"

Without thinking I said, "Okay."

She breathed a sigh of relief, "Thank you. We'll send you the 'Consent to Serve' forms."

After I hung up, I thought, "What did I just do? I'm already committed to be State Commander of the Disabled American Veterans Auxiliary—an organization to which I had belonged for nearly forty years. Bayside College is moving from a two year to a four year nursing program. We have major curriculum work ahead. I don't have time for this. I've got to call her back."

As I mulled it over, I recalled that the faculty of my basic nursing program had emphasized the importance of joining the professional organizations—the American Nurses Association (ANA) and the National League for Nursing. I'd maintained my dues in both organizations for nearly 34 years.

For several years my schedule didn't allow me to attend meetings or conventions on a regular basis. Occasionally I was able to attend an educational program or go to a convention on late Friday and stay over until the convention closed early Saturday.

In 1981 I attended the Annual Meeting of District 5. A former faculty member at Boston University School of Nursing encouraged me to join a committee. I joined the Nursing Practice Committee and became an active participant in the District. The earliest project that I participated in was the development of *An Application of the ANA Standards of Nursing Practice.*

Members of the Committee had solicited position descriptions and evaluation tools from various clinical settings in the District and used these to develop a protocol for applying the ANA Standards of Nursing Practice in Clinical Practice Settings. The Committee published its work and the publication was available through the District. Their work had an impact at the time on nursing practice in the area.

Later I was elected to a position on the state Cabinet for Nursing Ethics. One of our major projects was the development of Guidelines for the Ethical Dimensions of Public Policy. We published a pamphlet that was available through the state organization office and we presented an educational program on these

Guidelines at the state convention. Another major project involved writing a grant and presenting programs in communities throughout the state that provided communities with the guidelines that they needed to deal with the AIDS issue in the public schools. The intent was to provide communities with the tools for ethical decision-making but not to dictate what the decision would be.

One day Sally, the staff person, at the State Nurses Association office, asked me, "Do you think that your hometown would be interested?"

I thought it was a possibility. I contacted the Health Education Coordinator for my hometown public school system. I explained the program to her.

Initially Pam seemed very interested, and said, "My goal is to have condoms in every school by fall."

I explained our goals to her, "We are neither speaking for nor against the use of condoms. We are seeking to provide communities with a framework for ethical decision-making. Each community would use the framework to make its own decision."

Pam was no longer interested. I told Sally what had happened. She reaffirmed that our program was designed for communities that didn't have predetermined agendas.

When I became Chairperson of the Nursing Practice Committee, the committee turned its attention to discharge planning. Changes in reimbursement patterns by third party payers had resulted in earlier discharge of patients from inpatient settings and a need for increased services in homecare. Ann, the Continuing Care Coordinator at Children's Rehabilitation Center, was a valuable resource to our committee. Her years of experience resulted in a wealth of knowledge about the workings of the various homecare agencies that had sprung up to meet the emerging demands for homecare of patients. We developed a continuing education program and were able to persuade Ann to be one of the presenters.

As second vice president of the District I continued as Chairperson of the Nursing Practice Committee (with a waiver from the Board of Directors) until we were able to recruit a new chairperson. Usually we had two co-chairpersons. Finally we were able to find two members who would take on this task.

In the meantime I was no longer eligible to be a member of the Cabinet for Nursing Ethics but I'd been elected to the Cabinet for Nursing Research. Prior to my election to this cabinet, the members had revisited an earlier pamphlet on poster presentation and developed a new publication—***Getting the Word Out***.

We decided that it was time to revisit the Standards for Clinical Research. The outcome of our work was the publication—***Guidelines for Conducting Clinically based Research***. Both publications—***Getting the Word Out*** and ***Guidelines for Conducting Clinically based Research***—have been published and are available through the state nurses association.

The next project that we undertook was examining how we could facilitate the dissemination of nursing research findings. We were able to recruit a graduate nursing student for an internship. The Cabinet on Nursing Research and Mary Beth worked on developing a process for promoting nursing research as a way to increase public awareness of the contributions of nursing. An outcome of our effort was an entire issue of the State Newsletter devoted to nursing research.

In the meantime, the State Nurses Association was undergoing reorganization. Instead of having several Cabinets with elected members, they decided to have Issues Groups and Focus Groups. My second term on the Cabinet on Nursing Research was interrupted. Our work was incomplete.

This reorganization took place during my first term as President of the District. In late August, I'd met with the outgoing president who was a candidate of the State Nurses Association. I was still reeling from the untimely tragic death of my niece who had left two young children—an eighteen-month-old daughter and an almost seven-year-old son. Karen's brother had just died and she had recently learned that she had acquired two blood borne pathogens from a needle stick injury in the emergency room where she was employed.

The previous executive director and the associate director of the District had both resigned. The search committee had not yet selected a replacement but the Board of Directors had secured the services of an Interim Executive Director.

In October I assumed the position of District President; a few weeks later Karen became the State President. My initial responsibilities were to address the three goals of the Board of Directors.

The first was to determine that level of staffing that would be needed to carry out the work of the District. The second was to initiate a new search for a new executive director. The third was to oversee the upgrading of communications within the office (improve our office computers and get us online).

Rosemary our faithful secretary had been promoted to the position of Office Manager. Rosemary has been defined as "the Glue that holds the District Together." She has earned this designation one hundred fold. Without her support we wouldn't have survived the transition.

Although the Board of Directors recommended that the position of Executive Director be reduced from a 40-hour position to a 32-hour position, the Executive Director that we were able to hire was a go-getter who helped to facilitate the growth of our District to new heights. In addition she was able to rectify some of the problems in our office communications and develop a WEB Page. We were an association on the move. Unfortunately the State Nurses Association was on a countermove.

As president I had tried to remain active on the Nursing Practice Committee that had merged with the Nursing Education Committee a few years earlier. The newly formed Nursing Education and Practice Committee continued to be concerned with discharge planning but their concern had a more specific focus: the homeless population. They presented an excellent education program that was well attended by nurses in the area. An outgrowth of the educational program was the formation of a Homelessness Issues Group. This group developed a guide to the types of shelters in Boston and criteria for entry. This guide is an excellent resource for emergency room nurses.

The District also sponsored an annual program for graduating senior nursing students that was designed to support their transition from the nursing student to the practicing nurse role. The District expanded its support to novice nurses by forming a New Graduate Role Group.

As the District was experiencing new growth, the State Nurses Association was being catapulted into turmoil. A small contingent was advocating disaffiliation from the American Nurses Association. As a District we worked hard to insure that the membership was informed about the Pros and Cons of Affiliation versus Disaffiliation. Our goal was to provide information to the members so that they could make an informed decision. We were able to persuade the State Nurses Association to hold town meetings throughout the State. Attendance could have been better but it wasn't.

Although the issue was defeated at the State Convention, a special meeting was scheduled. After a long struggle, the small minority managed somehow to muster up enough members to vote for disaffiliation. The members of our district were disheartened. We investigated alternatives.

Ultimately a new affiliate of the American Nurses Association was formed and is in its initial growth phase. At some of our early meetings the Massachusetts Association for Registered Nurses (MARN) has addressed issues that are of concern to all practicing nurses.

This is a time of crisis for nursing that weighs heavily on the hearts of all of us in the nursing profession. As the population ages and the numbers of persons needing nursing services increases, the pool from which we draw applicants had been diminishing and the opportunities for this pool has expanded. Although we have had nursing shortages in the past, the current nursing shortage surpasses them. Unless the trend is reversed, the public is in trouble.

Several events have helped to reverse this trend. The American Nurses Association and other organizations have sponsored the Nursing Reinvestment Act—Legislation that would encourage young people to choose nursing as a career. The Johnson and Johnson Campaign to promote nurse recruitment through its discovernursing.com and public service announcements on the National Television Networks have been effective. Applications to nursing programs are on the rise.

The local constituent of the American Nurses Association was only one of several professional organizations to which I belonged and was active. These organizations played an important role in my professional development and in expanding my knowledge base for nursing practice and education. In addition I subscribed to numerous journals and attended an abundance of continuing education programs. I learned a lot about nursing but nothing prepared me to be a patient. I knew how to go about seeking the information I needed and the caregivers that I needed to go on the journey that had become so important.

10

Making Sure that the Enemy Never Returns

As preparations for chemotherapy began, I wondered how I would feel afterwards. Nausea has been so prevalent that women whom I knew shared stories of anticipatory nausea that appeared earlier and earlier during each progressive round of chemotherapy. They were dreadfully ill.

My sister-in-law agreed to take me to the Cancer Center each week. This wasn't easy for her. She had to take her granddaughter to kindergarten at 8:15 and pick her up at 11:15. Every 21days she' pick me up at 9:30 or 10:00 AM and drop me off at the Cancer Center for a 10:00 or 10:30 AM appointment. Six hours later she'd return for me. When she returned for me, she usually brought her granddaughter with her. Beforehand we had planned to have her granddaughter visit with her great-grandmother, but our plans were changed.

Having a variety of foods that were easy to prepare after a day of chemotherapy is important. I gathered quite an assortment: foods to eat in case I had constipation, foods to eat in case I had diarrhea, powdered milk that I could add to bottled milk to increase calories, and a ton of hard candy to relieve the soreness of mouth lesions. A supply of plastic utensils in case I experienced the metallic taste that Ricky mentioned was also needed.

Joanna looked at my wound on the 31st and verified that it was healed. The periodontist verified that my gums had healed after surgery. I called Ricky and told her that chemotherapy was a go! Then my stomach sank.

Before work on February 5th, I went to the cancer center for my initial blood work. At the time my CA 125 was 135—the highest that mine ever had been.

Some women have levels higher than 4000. My prognosis was good but I didn't know it.

After work we celebrated my niece's sixth birthday with pizza, cake, and ice cream and lots of presents. When I purchased her birthday outfits, I bought a little baseball suit for Sam. I felt that I owed him my life because he hung in there so that his mother could perform my life-saving surgery. Dr. D could've made arrangements for her mentor and partner to operate on me if it became necessary. I've heard good things about him but I'd developed a strong trust in Dr. D. I was relying on her to save my life. She did.

Two days later I started chemotherapy. I woke up very early and couldn't get back to sleep. I'd taken my medication the night before at 10:00 PM and in the morning at 9:00 AM. My sister-in-law was anxious. She arrived early. She's usually not early. My mother was crying, "I'll say a prayer for you." I knew that she would. She says a million prayers every day. A lot of folks are on her prayer list.

I grabbed my backpack and went out to the car. My sister-in-law told me that her friend's sister had died the evening before. She had been dying from cancer of the liver. The way that her sister explained it was that she had metastastic cancer of the liver but that they didn't know the primary source. I didn't understand this.

She asked, "Can you watch the kids while we go to the wake? And the funeral?" My nephew would go to school and come over after school. My niece would stay out of school while they went to the funeral. I could handle this.

We arrived at the Cancer Center. I grabbed my backpack and went in to the Reception Desk. Soon after my arrival, Cindy called my name. She introduced herself to me as my primary nurse. She gave me her card and told me that I would call her for symptom management.

She led me to the smaller of the two treatment areas and told me that I could choose any cubicle. She commented, "I like it back here because it is quieter." She set up the area for my comfort and hooked me up with a remote control and earphones so I could listen to my selections without disturbing anyone else.

After Cindy got me settled, she started an IV in my right arm. She started an intravenous medication running. Each time I came I received diphenhydramine and lorazepam. These medications were being given to prevent side effects of the chemotherapy medication. These medications could be given over 15–20 minutes. While she was calling for my first chemotherapy medication, a volunteer came in with a menu so that I could select lunch. I chose a tuna sandwich on rye, ginger ale, and tapioca pudding. Cindy returned with paclitaxel (Taxol)—my first chemotherapy medication. This medication was in a glass IV bottle. She and another nurse verified my name and the accuracy of the medication and dosage. She wore gloves to protect herself during handling of the medication and from blood borne pathogens. This is standard practice. She set the flow rate so that this medication would run in over three or four hours.

After the paclitaxel was absorbed, she started other medications—ondansetron and cimetidine. These were also being given to prevent side-effects of the chemotherapy medication. Cindy obtained the carboplatin (Paraplatin)—my second chemotherapy medication and took the same precautions. Cindy set the flow rate on the IV pump so that this medication would run in over 15–60 minutes.

According to the Davis Drug Guide for Nurses paclitaxel has its peak effect on white blood cell counts in 11 days and an effect lasting 21 days. Carboplatin has its peak effect on blood counts in 21 days and an effect lasting for 28 days. Common effects of the reduction in red cell counts, white cell counts, and platelets are fatigue, infection, and bleeding. Ricky's teaching had focused on prevention and early detection of these effects. The blood tests that monitored the actual cell counts before each round of chemotherapy were a necessary nuisance.

Before lunch I experienced some drowsiness that I attributed to my early awakening. The chemotherapy medications didn't trigger any undesirable side effects; diphenhydramine and lorazepam, medications that were used to control these side effects, had made me drowsy. Although the effects of diphenhydramine wore off in about four hours, the effects of lorazepam could last up to 48 hours. Having someone else drive me home after chemotherapy was crucial.

My day at the Cancer Center ended about 3:30 PM. Cindy gave me a schedule for my next visit that would be in three weeks. My sister-in-law brought me home. The children stayed for supper and spend a quiet evening with us. My brother came for them after the wake.

My niece arrived the next morning at 9:00 AM. She sat at the dining room table, looked at me and asked, "Well, Auntie, what do you have planned?"

I laughed, "Today's a school day. What's your school day usually like?"

She described a typical school day. "When we come in, we sit in a large circle, it's really an oval, and the teacher reads a story. Then we talk about the story. Then we do an activity. We do our numbers and then we have recess. Then we have snack and then we do our colors. Then she tells us what our homework is and we go home. When I get home, Grammy makes me lunch. Later I do my homework."

Now we had a plan. We selected some books, gathered our supplies, and set out to work. First we read a story. She pointed out words that she knew and words that she didn't know.

When it was time to do numbers, she showed me how her teacher writes problems and how she and the other children do their sums. This was easy.

The weather was pleasant and we went outside for recess. She taught me how to play soccer. Six-year-olds devise their own rules and explain them as they make them up. She loved running after the ball. I live on a main street so I had one rule. She couldn't run after the ball if it rolled out of the yard.

After recess, we returned to our "classroom for a day" and had a snack. We talked about healthy food choices. She decided to draw a picture of a healthy snack and label each item. She knows the food guide pyramid and makes good food choices.

When it was time to do our colors, she told me that her teacher was teaching the class some Spanish words. We looked through a book with pictures that were labeled in Spanish and English for a topic. She wanted to learn colors in Spanish by playing "I am thinking of something that is (say color)." We learned the colors of the rainbow in Spanish: rojo (red), anaranjado (orange), amarillo (yellow), verde (green), azul (blue), morado (purple), negro (black), y blanco (white).

Dismissal time was approaching. As teacher I had to make up some home-work. I assigned some problems and some spelling words. After lunch she did her homework. She stapled her papers together and put them in her backpack. She planned to show them to her teacher on Monday.

I went to the hairdresser the following day and asked her to cut my hair short—very short! Although I'd always worn my hair short, I wasn't used to wearing it straight. Some of the senior nursing students actually liked my new hairstyle. I said, "Don't get too used to it. I won't have it for long."

Exactly two weeks after my first round of chemotherapy as I combed my hair, the first few strands started to fall out as Ricky had predicted. All I could say is "Oh, damn! I'm not going to defy the odds."

The following evening my colleagues at District 5 MNA went to dinner. I wore a wig for the first time. Very little hair had fallen out but I was afraid that hair would fall into my colleague's food. They might not think that this was too cool.

Some of my colleagues didn't know that I had ovarian cancer. I had purposely kept things low key while efforts to maintain affiliation with the American Nurses Association were underway. I didn't want those who were spearheading the disaffiliation movement to know that I was vulnerable.

Rosanna asked, "How are you doing?" Her question elicited questions and expressions of concern. Their concerns were easily allayed as I looked well. I enjoyed the evening immensely but I was up early the next day.

My niece came by to spend the weekend so that my brother and his wife could celebrate their anniversary. In anticipation of my rapidly changing hairstyle I tried to prepare her for the inevitable. I explained, "The medicine that I'm taking to make me better will make my hair fall out. Lots of hair will fall out today. It'll grow back in time for your grandfather's birthday on the third of July."

After staring strangely at me for a minute, she commented in disbelief, "That's really stupid."

I agreed, "Yes it is, but it's going to happen. Wait and see."

I decided to comb my hair often so that it wouldn't fall out everywhere. This approach seemed to work.

My niece asked, "Could I do that?" After I gave her the go-ahead, she combed out hair periodically throughout the day. She really enjoys combing other people's hair so it was fun for her. It was unsettling for me.

In anticipation of my second round of chemotherapy, I went to the Cancer Center on February 25th for blood work and an examination by Dr. Schwartz. After a thorough history and examination, he told me, "You had a dramatic decrease in your CA 125 after your initial therapy. This is what we like to see. You seem to be doing okay so far." I agreed.

When I opened the door to my mother's house the next day, I heard her calling for help. I couldn't see her at first because the dining room table blocked my view. She was kneeling in the kitchen. She had fallen and was trying to make her way to the telephone so that she could call for help. She might've made it if the kitchen floor of her old house hadn't been an inch lower than the dining room floor. Getting up over a slight rise was too much for her.

Because of my recent surgery, I couldn't help her up. I called 911. The responding Emergency Medical Technicians lifted her into a chair and insisted that she would be okay. I repeatedly told them that she had landed on her hip and needed to be checked at the emergency room. I couldn't believe how hard I had to work to convince them to take her to the Emergency Room. I couldn't believe that they didn't make this assessment on their own. The way that she described her fall suggested that she might have injured her hip. She needed to be checked out.

She had fractured her right hip and was admitted to the hospital. The orthopedist on call didn't come in that evening. I was upset when I went home because I didn't know when her hip would be repaired.

I came into the hospital very early the next day. The orthopedist had already seen my mother and was planning to repair her hip imminently. I recognized him because he had set my fractured wrist on Christmas Day 1995. When I told him who I was, he said, "Walk with me to the operating room and I'll explain what I'm planning to do on the way."

After they took her into surgery, I went home to rest. They were transferring her from the post anesthesia care unit (PACU) to her room when I returned. She came through the surgery very well.

During her hospital stay she was diagnosed with diabetes mellitus. This created havoc as they attempted to regulate her blood sugar. The fractured hip would've been enough. She didn't need the additional stress. Neither did I.

I was relieved that her surgery was over before my next chemotherapy in the morning. After a long day I went home and "crashed".

My sister-in-law picked me up at 9:30 AM the next day and brought me to the Cancer Center where I had my second round of chemotherapy. Cindy called me in and carried out my chemotherapy. Considering all that had happened this week, my chemotherapy went well.

The medications that they give to prevent the unwelcome effects of the therapeutic medications made me drowsy. Although I brought journals to read, I wasn't able to focus. Instead I watched boring TV programs. I arrived too late to make a menu selection. The volunteer had remembered my food choices and placed an order for me. I appreciated him remembering and bringing me what I would've ordered.

After lunch I was able to do some reading. My sister-in-law and the children came for me at 3:30 PM. My chemotherapy ended at 3:40 PM. While they waited for me, the children acquainted themselves with the occupants of the aquarium. Whenever they came to the cancer center they liked to make sure that every fish was present and accounted for and to look for newcomers.

We went to visit my mother for a while. When we arrived they were helping her back into bed after a very brief walk. She looked worn. I thought, "We're in this for the long haul. Will she ever regain her former independence?" Seeing the impact of the fall and the surgery on her spirit was disheartening.

When I arrived the next day March 1st I was pleased to learn that the discharge coordinator was optimistic. She recommended three potential placements for my mother. I met with the admission coordinator of one facility and arranged a visit later that day. I called the second facility and arranged a visit as well. I never contacted the third facility.

The admissions coordinator from the Shaunessey Kaplan Rehabilitation Hospital (SKRH) was optimistic that my mother would be accepted. She told me, "Your mother reminds me of my mother." Because of the newly diagnosed diabetes she wasn't sure which unit that she would be assigned to. I was sure that she would do her best to assure my mother's admission.

I hoped that the program at SKRH would not be too intensive for my mother but I knew that the program at the other facility wouldn't be adequate. I briefed my brother on my findings. My brother, an auto mechanic, said, "I'll yield to your judgment on this." When I suggested the program at SKRH to my mother, she asked, "What does your brother think?" I groaned, "Dear God, this is medical care, not a car." Before I left the hospital for the day, the discharge coordinator said that the discharge was tentatively set for Monday but could happen over the weekend.

I was very tired when I went home. I slept late Saturday. At 11:00 AM I got a call from the hospital. The ambulance was coming to take my mother to SKRH at 12:30 PM. I barely made it to the hospital in time for her departure.

The ambulance drivers took my mother and I took her belongings and headed out. Although they pulled out of the hospital parking lot before me, I arrived at SKRH first. I awaited her arrival. I wondered what was delaying them.

While I was waiting one of the aides spoke to me. Her husband is a member of the Disabled American Veterans—an organization in which both my mother and I've been very active for over 40 years. She looked after my mother and kept me posted on her progress whenever I visited.

After her arrival the admitting nurse conducted a thorough nursing history and assessment. The process tired my mother and she needed to rest afterwards.

Meanwhile, I looked at a sign at her bedside that listed Joanne A. as the program director. At the time I didn't realize that I knew her.

My mother was settled in and needed rest. So did I. I went home.

That evening my feet bothered me. This shouldn't be surprising because I had been active for the last few days. No matter what I did, I wasn't comfortable. If I rested my feet on the sofa, I was miserable. I placed a pillow under each leg to lift my feet off the sofa. It helped a little.

Ricky had suggested glutamine three times a day. Glutamine is available in caplets or powder. I took one dose—ten large caplets—after the first round of chemotherapy. The amount of water that it took to swallow ten large caplets was too much for me. Glutamine powder can be mixed in milk or juice. I could take the powder but it didn't help. Although Ricky had told me that acetaminophen and ibuprofen wouldn't help, I decided to try them. They didn't help.

Later, Rosanna (my colleague who had ovarian cancer) told me my discomfort was related to peripheral neuritis. She told me that the Vitamin B 6 should help. I'd been taking Vitamin B 6 50 mg three times a day as recommended. When I learned that slow release tablets were available, I decided to take one in the morning and one in the evening.

I spoke to Rita after church on March 9th. I told her about my mother's fall. She promised to pray for her recovery. She commented, "I heard that you had a little minor surgery yourself." When I told Rita about the extent of my surgery, she shared her story with me. I had been aware that Rita had cancer since 1980 but I didn't know the details. Now I know that Rita is a real survivor!

> Rita said, "I had ovarian cancer 34 years ago (1968). I was in stage 3. In those days they used nitrogen mustard and radiation."
>
> I said, "Oh, I didn't realize that you had ovarian cancer. I didn't know what kind you had."
>
> She continued, "You know, my daughter is a nurse. She has a friend who is at Sloan Kettering. She told her that I had ovarian cancer back then. Her friend wanted to know, 'When did your mother die?' She was surprised when my daughter said that I was still living."

Later I learned that while her daughter was at the University of Pennsylvania, she had a fellowship at Sloan Kettering. Her associates at Sloan Kettering were surprised to learn that her mother had survived ovarian cancer stage 3 in 1968.

Later Rita also told me, "You know, one of the things that my daughter said to me is, "They don't really know how to manage the pain." I was able to tell Rita that pain management protocols have improved remarkably and that people with cancer need to tell their caretakers if their pain isn't being relieved."

Rita went on to reminisce about her experiences on the maternity unit at the local hospital. "I still remember when you used to come in and take care of me. You and Lois were the only two who talked to us. We so appreciated it."

My conversation with Rita benefited me in many ways. First I knew that she would include my mother and me in her prayers. Second I had met a real ovarian cancer survivor. If she survived, I had more hope than I had realized. Finally her affirmation of the support that I had given her when she had her children lifted my spirits at a time when I was undergoing a lot of stress in my professional life.

I always enjoyed my associations with Lois. She was assistant head nurse when I first arrived at the local hospital. She was an unofficial lactation consultant before anyone ever heard of them. She taught me a lot about helping women who were trying to breastfeed at a time when so few women did and so little support existed. In spite of the paucity of knowledge about how to help mothers breastfeed, she did her best to help. I found it very rewarding when I could help a woman get her infant off to a good start. Later she became the maternity supervisor.

When I graduated from my first nursing program, Lois made a beautiful ceramic nurse for me. It is one of my treasures. When I saw Lois recently, she lamented, "We did everything wrong in those days." I said, "No, we did the best that we knew and we provided the only support that the women received. We did have some successes. Others learned from what we did and built on our successes."

On Monday I received a voice mail from Joanne A. She said, "You don't know me but I am the program director at SKRH. I wanted to let you know that we have rounds on Tuesdays at 1:30 PM and family members are welcome to attend." As I listened to her message, I recognized her voice. Joanne A. had been one of my nursing students at Bayside College several years earlier.

When I spoke with her, Joanne was surprised to learn that I remembered her and that a colleague and I often wondered what she and others in the program were doing. She proved to be a very helpful advocate. When she learned of my health status, she emphasized the importance of my mother being relatively independent so I could provide her care at home.

Over the next few weeks my mother had her ups and downs but she made slow steady progress. I had some fatigue but I attributed it to the combination of my work schedule and my visiting her after work.

While I was visiting my mother a neuropsychologist came in to assess my mother's cognitive status. He told jokes to decide if she could explain them. An example would be: "Why is six afraid of seven? Because 7–8–9!" She got every joke but she didn't think they were that funny. She thought that he needed some new material. She asked me to bring in some of the joke books that she received from the Federation for the Blind. I did.

My mother was 87 years old on March 15th. The family arranged to celebrate her birthday at SKRH. My plan was to bring her to the family room on the fifth floor so that we wouldn't disturb her roommate.

When I arrived with sandwiches and party goods, she was already in bed. This was the earliest that she had gone to bed since she was admitted. Her roommate wasn't in the room and her bed was unmade. Her daughter who was usually there from daybreak to nightfall wasn't there. My mother said, "She was gone when I returned from therapy. No one will answer my questions. I don't think she's coming back." The fact that her bed was unmade surprised me. If she were coming back, her bed should be ready.

Our family began to arrive. The children were ravenously hungry. I gave my niece a cup of soda and a chicken kabob sub and a napkin on a plate and suggested, "Sit over here on the floor. Let's pretend that we are at a picnic."

When the others saw that it worked for my niece, those who didn't have chairs joined her on the floor. I overheard my niece say to her aunt, "Isn't this the most fun you ever had?"

I breathed a sign of relief. The party would be a success. We had a great time. My mother got a lot of plants. This was okay. She loves plants. I would have something to do when I visited—water plants and then water more plants.

My sister-in-law had brought birthday cakes and candles. After we sang "Happy Birthday", my nephew helped her to blow out the candles. Soon the party was over.

While my mother was saying good bye to everyone who had come to her party, her roommate arrived on a stretcher. The staff came running in to make up her bed. Her daughter told us, "They took her to surgery to fix repair a broken shoulder." My mother and I were relieved to know that she was okay.

Her daughter who usually ate with her mother had missed supper. We still had food and were able to provide her with a substantial meal and birthday cake. She appreciated our kindness. After that she provided me with updates on my mother's progress whenever I came in.

On March 20th I went in for my blood work and for an examination with Jean, the nurse practitioner who was filling in for Ricky who was on vacation. When I signed in, I saw a friend. Although I knew that she had cancer, she hadn't spoken directly to me about it.

She did tell my mother about her cancer but my mother had a hearing problem and didn't have the details. As a nurse, I respect privacy—something other people in the group to which we belong did not seem to value as much. I waited for her to share her story with me.

When she realized why I was there, she asked, "Why didn't you call me?"

I learned that Dr S was her oncologist and Ricky was her nurse practitioner. She loved them both. So did I. Having caring, compassionate, and competent health care providers helps ease the burden of the unwanted journey.

I told her that I didn't share my illness with anybody in the group because they share private information in their public newsletter. Today she shared her story with me. She told me that she had a beta cell lymphoma. She was here today for laboratory work and a medication to stimulate her red blood cells, as they were very low.

I asked, "Epoetin? Procrit?"

She responded, "Yes. I'm anemic." She appeared very pale and exhausted!

I saw her less often at meetings and other events but we kept track of each other's progress.

I had my third round of chemotherapy the next day. Michelle came to the waiting area to get me. She explained that Cindy was ill. I was concerned because Cindy was expecting a baby in September. My confidence in Michelle was already established. In January she had checked my veins and assured me that I had several access sites and could receive chemotherapy IV. She was okay with me!

The next morning was a gorgeous spring day. It was good to be able to go outside to do yard work and get exercise. I may have been a little too enthusiastic.

I was tired on Saturday but I had work to do. I was trying to anchor the rugs so that my mother wouldn't trip when she got home. I was also trying to set up the durable medical equipment that she would need at home. They didn't bring the walker that she needed. I had to make calls and locate the one she could use at another Medical Supply Company.

My mother was discharged on Good Friday March 29th. The visiting nurse would be in on Saturday and the physical therapist would be in on Monday. My brother planned to meet me there with his van. I still had things to do to get her home ready for her. I was a few minutes late.

Although I had already brought as much as I could home the day before, she still had a lot of stuff to take out to the car. When we got her outside, she knew exactly how to move from the wheelchair into the van. She was just too short. I discovered a metal case in the back of my brother's van. It was the perfect size and shape to serve as a step stool. She moved into the van easily.

The neuropsychologist who'd seen my mother a few weeks earlier came outside to say "Good Bye." She was glad to see him. She asked me to get the Joke Books out of the car. He read a few jokes out loud. He was pleasantly surprised, "These are perfect!"

I had to make one more stop for medical supplies. My brother arrived with my mother before me and was waiting for me to help her out of the van and into the house. She was happy to be home.

The VNA nurse came in and conducted an assessment on Saturday. The initial assessment is lengthy because Medicare requires an Outcomes Assessment (OASIS). The nurse planned to visit every other day until the wound had healed substantially. Then, she would turn over responsibility for the wound to me.

The physical therapist came in on Monday and conducted an assessment. Prior to discharge I had completed a form that had provided them with information from the number of steps that she had to climb to get in the house to a detailed layout of her home. It was complete and they didn't need to make a home visit prior to her discharge. She planned to visit one day a week and asked if a student could come on a second day. This arrangement continued until my mother no longer needed physical therapy. My mother continued to use a walker until August.

When I mentioned that I had seen a four pronged cane at a yard sale, she said, "Oh, Aunt Anna had one. I could use one of those." I went to the Medical Supply Company and bought a four pronged cane. Gradually she began to use it. After a transition period she no longer used the walker. Recently someone suggested that she get a walker, as a mutual acquaintance seemed to be getting around with one. My mother commented, "I used to use one. I have graduated to a cane." She was pleased with her progress. Her hip is fully healed but she still uses the cane because of a preexisting knee condition.

As I headed toward the Cancer Center and my visit with Dr. S on April 8th, I mulled over everything that had happened since my last visit with him prior to my mother's fall.

A woman whom I had known from church in the 1950s and 1960s was in front of me. I hadn't seen her for several years and wouldn't have recognized her if I didn't hear her say her name.

When I spoke to her, she seemed to recall who I was. After I signed in, I went to obtain a specimen and take it to the laboratory. She'd already been called in to see her physician when I returned to the waiting area. I read her obituary in the local newspaper a few weeks later. I wouldn't see her again at the Cancer Center.

After a thorough history and examination Dr. S assured me that I was making good progress. This news was heartening!

When my sister-in-law picked me up on April 11th, to take me to chemotherapy, she looked at my backpack and exclaimed, "You always look as if you are going to camp." My fourth round of chemotherapy went smoothly. Cindy was back to work and was doing well. She was worried about going into the hospital to give birth. We talked about what would happen. I gave her my number in case she wanted to call me with more questions.

On April 16th I saw my downtown doctor for the first time since her son's early and welcome arrival. While I was waiting for her, I observed four women come one after the other and take seats beside each other in the waiting area. A nurse came to call one of them. She smiled and said, "I see that the Tuesday club is here."

The four women had met each other at the Cancer Center and had decided to schedule their chemotherapy at the same time. I thought, "What a support group! I never saw the same people twice when I came in."

While I was watching the fourth woman go into the day hospital area, a member of my parish came in with her brother in law. When she saw me she called out and asked, "Terry, are you here for yourself or did you come with someone?"

I turned to see who was talking to me. I told her my story. She told me that she was bringing her brother-in-law in because the person who usually brings him was on vacation.

She promised to remember me in her prayers. She is a minister of communion and a faithful member of our parish. I am grateful to be added to her prayer list.

Things are moving along. I went in for laboratory work and a visit with Ricky on April 30th. She questioned me in detail about the peripheral neuritis that was still plaguing me. She asked, "How bad is it? This is the only reason to reduce the dose. We really don't want to do this."

I responded, "It's a nuisance but a tolerable one." It didn't occur to me that she was planning to recommend a change in one of my medications.

Two days later I received my fifth round of chemotherapy. Within the next few days I felt as if I had had a double whammy. After I had finished chemotherapy and reviewed my medical records, I learned that I had actually received a lower dose.

While I was undergoing chemotherapy, I had a prearranged interview at Cancer Center for a research study that was investigating Ovarian Cancer Tumor Risk. The study that was being conducted by the Dana Farber Cancer Center was looking at diet, medical and family history. As I looked at the study protocol, my own theory about ovarian cancer came to mind.

> The changes that I had made in my diet took place prior to the targeted date in this study. Discussing my earlier diet might have explained my risk better. It was difficult to respond to the interview questions within the framework of their study, but I did. I was looking at the study from the perspective of the researcher. I had a hard time looking at the study from the other side of the looking glass.

> While I was a student at the University of Rhode Island, I had completed a questionnaire for a classmate's study. She was working in conjunction with the Cancer Prevention Research Center in 1991. Her study focused on practices that people engage in with regard to the amount of fat in their diet and what they do to reduce the amount of fat in their diet. At this time my dietary practices were very different. I was trying to reduce overall calories but I was not trying to limit overall fat or animal fat as I now do.

My niece spent the weekend of May 4th and 5th with us. The worse effects of chemotherapy that I had experienced surfaced. When she asked me to play hopscotch with her, she hopped and I walked. Each time she hopped skillfully, I praised her achievements and rewarded her.

I would say, "You did so well that you get an extra turn—two turns to my one, then three turns to my one. Soon she was getting eight turns to my one. She caught on to what I was doing but she also knew that I was very tired. She was happy to have someone to play with.

That evening, she wanted to play a game with me, but I needed to lie down for awhile. At my mother's suggestion, she lay down beside me on the living room couch. After resting about 15 minutes, we played "Chutes and Ladders" and "Candy Land."

Late Monday evening May 6th I received a call from Dr. P—a physician at Massachusetts General. He was on his way home from a long day at the hospital and he was calling me on his cell phone. As he went through the Sorrow Drive underpasses his voice faded in and out and I had difficulty understanding him. He was trying to tell me about a clinical trial that he thought might interest me. The clinical trial involved a new treatment for women with ovarian cancer. If I was interested, the study involved surgery and being randomized to an experimental or a control group. My physician could do the surgery if I decided to enter the study.

The clinical trial had an acronym but I didn't grasp it at first. I had difficulty figuring out the sequence of events in the clinical trial because I missed parts of the conversation and had to ask him to repeat portions of his explanation. His call aroused anxiety. I wondered, "What did they find in my blood studies? Has my condition changed? Why is he calling me?"

I played e-mail tag with Dr. D and voice-mail tag with Dr. P and finally obtained clarity about the study. Dr. D explained that it was a Phase III clinical trial. She emphasized that if I wanted to consider taking part in this clinical trial that I had to make an appointment with Dr. P to discuss it. She was adamant that it was my decision.

Understanding the distinction between Phase I trials, Phase II trials, and Phase III trials prior to taking part in a clinical study is important. During phase I an initial dose based on animal testing is given to participants who agree to take part in the clinical trial. The dose is increased and then reduced until a safe effective dose with minimal toxicity is determined. During phase II the established dose of the drug is given to patients who meet the criteria for entry into the study to find out if the drug is effective in this group. During Phase III patients who agree to take part in the study are randomized to either receive the new drug or to receive the standard treatment. The purpose is to determine if the new treatment is more effective than the treatment already in place. When the findings are known, other factors, such as relative cost and toxicity, help to determine whether the new treatment is approved for use.

The new treatment that he was describing had already been tested. A safe effective dose had been settled. Now they were comparing the proposed treatment with standard practice. Inasmuch as this clinical trial was a randomized study, I had a fifty-fifty chance of being assigned to either the new treatment or standard practice.

When I went in to see Dr. P on May 13th, he explained the SMART Study and gave me the seven-page consent form and a copy of the four-page patient leaflet. He also gave me a copy of a twelve-page consent form of a Phase II clinical trial that was being done with women who had confirmed residual disease.

I agreed to consider the SMART Study and let him know by the following week whether I would take part in this clinical trial. I also told him that I wasn't able to think about the other clinical trial. If Dr D were to find residual disease during laparoscopy, I don't know if I would have reconsidered.

I promised Andrea that I would fax the consent to her after I met with my oncologist at the Cancer Center. Andrea coordinated several aspects of the study. I wanted to get a sense of how my oncologists felt about the clinical trial before I signed on.

The SMART (Study of Monoclonal Antibody Radioimmune Therapy) Study is a clinical trial. Clinical trials don't come with guarantees. Risks and benefits are explained and need to be weighed by study participants. Decisions are based on this process.

The SMART Study *could* be beneficial if undetected residual cells had been left behind during my original surgery and if chemotherapy wasn't effective in destroying those cells. If I didn't enter the clinical trial, recurrence or relapse was a possibility. I had already decided that if I had a relapse I would agree to aggressive therapy whatever that meant. My decision to enter the clinical trial was based on my realization that my participation would be proactive whereas chemotherapy after relapse would be reactive. I knew that I could be part of the control group but I also could be part of the treatment group.

Graduation at Bayside College was held on Saturday. For the first time in nine years it rained. It had been raining very hard all night. Some areas of the campus had flooded in the past. Yet, the powers that be didn't possess the wisdom to move the ceremony inside.

The maintenance staff had placed a piece of plywood over a small river that had emerged overnight and they supported us as we walked over the bridge to the outdoor tent. Our feet were relatively dry until we entered the tent where the water was a few inches deep.

I wore heavy clothing underneath my academic regalia and a plastic hooded cape over it. I was able to remove the cape when we got inside. I was probably the only dry person in the whole tent. Although it was cold and damp, the weather didn't bother me. The young woman who sat next to me has a chronic illness. She was shivering throughout the ceremony. Her shivering concerned me. I asked her if she wanted to go inside but she didn't want to.

The college had planned an outdoor dedication to the new library wing after the graduation. It was cancelled. Usually the reception for the graduates and their families after graduation has typically been a delightful event. I decided to forego this event.

Blood work and an appointment with Dr S were scheduled on May 20th. When he saw me, Dr. S said, "I'm glad that you decided to take part in the trial." Sensing no hesitancy on his part, I signed the consent form and faxed it to MGH. This set a sequence of activities into motion. These will be discussed in the next chapter.

When I mentioned the persistent peripheral neuritis, Dr. S said, "It may never go away." It never did. While I was undergoing chemotherapy, it seemed to be worse from Saturday evening through Sunday evening. Then it subsided somewhat. Although it didn't disappear after I completed chemotherapy, it is a minor nuisance in the larger scheme of things. I had my life back and a promising future. I knew that oncologists couldn't always be optimistic but my growing team of oncologists and oncology nurses seemed to be optimistic, even if somewhat guardedly, about my prognosis.

The college traditionally celebrated the end of each year with a day of fun for the faculty and staff. This year they decided to offer the opportunity to go on a whale watch. I woke up to a beautiful but cool spring day. I put on layers of heavy clothing, a hat, scarf, and gloves, and headed to Gloucester. Although I took a wrong turn and landed at the wrong dock, the people in the office called their competitors. After verifying where I should be, they provided me with directions.

I made it to the boat just in time. I joined a few acquaintances on deck and chatted with them. While we were still in Gloucester harbor, the weather was cool but pleasant.

Shortly after the boat pulled out of the harbor, the captain announced that whales and dolphins had been spotted on the starboard side. I watched the whales and dolphins in their natural habitat for a short while. As the boat moved further from shore, the ocean breezes became cooler and cooler. I started to shiver. I located a seat inside where the wind didn't blow and spent the rest of the whale watch inside. I tried to venture outside later but it was still too cold for me. My choices were shivering or seclusion. I choose seclusion.

I had my annual mammogram on May 22nd. Having one type of cancer doesn't confer immunity against other types of cancer. The report was good.

The following day I had my final chemotherapy. The chemotherapy was uneventful. While I was there, the social worker provided me with information about a support group and promised to send me a newsletter that is available to women with ovarian cancer. She kept her promise. Completing chemotherapy was cause for celebration.

Everyone who has ovarian cancer soon becomes aware of acquaintances who had ovarian cancer or who have friends or relatives who have ovarian cancer. Ten of eleven nurses on the Board of Directors of a professional nursing organization where I served as President are women. Two of the ten women had had ovarian cancer. I became the third. We are doing well.

The secretary of another professional nursing organization where I serve as a director told me that her brother's wife had ovarian cancer. Her disease had been diagnosed in the third stage and she did poorly. After her death her brother wanted to know, "Why didn't they do tests? Why didn't they discover this earlier?" Although I could explain that the available tests weren't definitive, this information isn't comforting when a loved one is affected. A woman from my church who was diagnosed with ovarian cancer in 1964 was also in the third stage. She is a quiet but real survivor.

Why did one woman diagnosed in the third stage die and another survive? I don't know. Ovarian cancer isn't a single disease. Ovarian cancer is a cluster of thirty diseases. Some types are worse than others.

My plans on May 25th were to join Irma and Sister B for lunch. The three of us had jointly coordinated the Religious Education Program in our parish for several years. After Sister B had been assigned to another parish, we met for lunch twice a year. I briefly considered canceling our lunch meeting after feeling light-headed for a split second. Then I decided to go. We had an enjoyable time.

When we got out our calendars to set another date, Sister B had a sense of urgency about having lunch again during the summer. She didn't give a reason. "I'd like to meet sooner rather than wait until after Christmas."

I was hesitant. I wasn't sure how I would respond to radioimmune therapy. Radioimmune therapy could affect my bone marrow. My bone marrow hadn't recovered from chemotherapy. I thought that I would be okay by the end of the summer. I suggested late August. Today would the last time that the three of us would have lunch together. A long-standing tradition would come to a screeching halt.

11

Seeking out the Hiding Places

After I faxed the signed consent form for the SMART Study to Andrea, a whole series of events were set into motion. This study had a strict timeframe. A CT Scan and laboratory work is scheduled three to four weeks after the final round of chemotherapy. If a tentative diagnosis of remission is supported, a laparoscopy is done to provide a more definitive diagnosis of remission.

If I were found to be in remission after laparoscopy, I'd be eligible for the study. Dr. D would be advised of the outcome of my random assignment and take the necessary steps to insure that I'd either receive radioimmune therapy or I'd receive standard treatment. I was randomly assigned to the experimental group. This meant that she'd leave a catheter in place so that I could receive Radioimmune Therapy.

The Cancer Center held a Cancer Survivor's Day Celebration on June 1st. It was my first time attending. I was baffled when the woman asked me, "How long have you been a survivor?"

She asked, "When were you diagnosed?"

I responded, "January 11th" (the day of my surgery). She gave me a badge that said I was a six-month survivor.

Things were in full swing when I arrived. The affair included a variety of activities, entertainment, making ice cream sundaes, and prizes. The nurses who had given me my chemotherapy were there and asked me how I was doing. I mentioned the upcoming clinical trial.

A large crowd was gathered around one table. People were making squares for a quilt in memory of loved ones. A woman was making a square in memory of her mother. I recognized her as the sister of a high school friend and a former neighbor. She told me that she was also a cancer survivor and had been treated at the Cancer Center. We took some pictures to send to her sister.

The CT scan was booked for June 11th. Dr D had told me that I might have a CT Scan a year after my surgery. Having the CT Scan sooner was a mixed blessing. I could know sooner that nothing else showed up but it might provide false reassurance if it was too soon for anything to show up.

When I arrived in radiology I observed that they had a new CT Scanner—one that was much less confining than the Scanner that they had used in November. The procedure went well and I was soon on my way home.

On June 20th the necessary blood work that would determine my eligibility to take part in the clinical trial was done. The blood work couldn't be done any earlier or any later. As soon as I had the blood drawn, I headed to the Disabled American Veterans State Convention in Marlborough. We had a busy and enjoyable weekend.

Four days later I had my first medical examination after finishing chemotherapy. In contrast to his initial gentle probing of my abdomen during my early postoperative days, Dr. S probed deeply into my abdomen. He did a thorough clinical breast examination and searched for but didn't find bad nodes anywhere. I was sure that if anything were there, he would've found it. Dr. S said, "Everything looks good!" So far, it's a go!

My preoperative visit was scheduled on June 26th. I went to the Cox Center at 9:30 AM to see Dr. D. Joanna, Andrea, and Laura joined us. They introduced Laura, the nurse practitioner who would be contacting me with the results of my laboratory work while I was in the SMART Study. This festive occasion seemed more like a reunion than a visit to a renowned physician's office—so much so that Dr. D had to remind the merrymakers that she needed to review the procedure and obtain consent for surgery.

After the merrymakers settled down, Dr. D got to do her part. She asked me if I knew what she would be doing. When she realized that I had a vague sense of what laparoscopy was, she said, "I am going to talk to you as if you don't know anything about it." She did.

This is an excellent approach. Physicians and nurses always know a lot about their own line of work but very little about what physicians or nurses in other areas do. Her explanation was simple and to the point. I already knew this, but I still needed to hear it from her. It was happening to me—not to somebody else.

Dr. D was very concerned about the potential complications of laparoscopy. I knew that these were hemorrhage, infection, and perforation. (HIP). She said, "We go in blind. In case of perforation I'm going to order a bowel prep. If anything were to happen, I want to be able to go in right away and fix it."

What she was saying made sense but I thought that she was talking about the standard preoperative prep that I'd undertaken in January. A surprise was in store for me.

Dr. D was also concerned about the remote possibility that she might find something. She said, "If I find something, I'm going to put in a port so I can give you intraperitoneal (into the belly) chemotherapy."

I knew that this would've happened if I had advanced disease at the time of my initial surgery. I knew that relapse was a possibility. Listening to her discussing the possibility that she was considering putting in the port was both unsettling and reassuring. It was scary thinking about the fact that as a person with cancer I needed to be aware that relapse or recurrence was always a possibility. It was good to know that Dr. D had a plan to set in motion in case of the worst case scenario instead of the best case scenario.

Dr. D continued, "I'm going to add this here (write 'IP port' on the consent form)." She did.

After I signed the consent form, we said our "Good Byes" and I went for my preoperative testing.

Preoperative testing was similar to my earlier visit prior to general surgery. In spite of the fact that a laparoscopy (viewing with a scope through a small incision) is generally less invasive than general surgery, the staff in the preoperative screening area does not skimp on services.

It went much easier for me this time because I had my blue card and I didn't need to stop at every restroom in the hospital complex. My entry into this study gave me special immunity. No one could offer me an opportunity to be a participant in other clinical trials. I was home for lunch.

A few hours later Jay the scheduling coordinator called me to tell me what time I was scheduled. She asked, "Did they give you the instructions for the bowel prep?"

I answered, "No, I thought that she wanted me to do the same thing that I did when I had the surgery."

She replied, "I think that she wants more than that."

I commented, "I didn't think it got any worse."

She replied, "Oh, yes it does. If you don't hear back from me, do what you did."

The following day I received the instructions for the bowel prep. The scheduling coordinator was right. It was worse!

My procedure had been scheduled originally for 8:00 AM and I was expected to arrive at 6:30 AM. I arranged transportation but I was concerned that my nephew who would be taking me home wouldn't be able to come for me until 5:30 PM. I didn't mind hanging out but I wasn't sure that the staff would want me lingering around.

Jay called me back to say that my procedure had been rescheduled for 1:00 PM with an arrival time of 12:00 noon. She said, "Don't worry about rushing. As the day goes on, surgeries tend to get backlogged." I was relieved to know that I wouldn't be waiting around too long for my nephew after all.

The bowel prep that Jay told me about allowed me to drink see-through liquids from Friday midnight through Sunday at midnight and then nothing to drink from midnight Sunday until after surgery.

My day on Sunday was spent alternating taking Neomycin and Erthromycin (antibiotics) and drinking Fleet's phosphosoda midmorning and midafternoon. My evening was spent capping this delightful experience off with a series of Fleet enemas.

Phosphosoda is gross. I drank it quickly. This was a mistake. I didn't retain it all. Nonetheless, the disgusting potion did its work. Its purpose is to empty the gut and empty the gut it did. The antibiotics would destroy the bacteria that normally live in the gut.

This prep would be very beneficial if my gut were perforated. Although I know that it could happen, I wasn't worried. The precautions that Dr. D was taking were reassuring. In the meantime I knew that I needed to learn how to tolerate Phosphosoda in the future. It is the bowel prep of choice prior to colonoscopy and other such delightful procedures.

I had the wisdom to postpone my colonoscopy that had been scheduled for July 3rd. The complications for colonoscopy are the same as the complications for laparoscopy: hemorrhage, infection, and perforation (HIP). It would've been an unwelcome problem if I spilled a radioactive substance in the endoscopy suite.

I was up and ready to roll in plenty of time to arrive at ambulatory surgery at MGH on July 1st. A snafu in my transportation arrangements resulted in my arrival at 12:40 and a change in the schedule.

The staff prepared me for the procedure. They gave me the typical gown, pajama bottoms, robe, and skid-proof slippers in exchange for my worldly possessions. I asked if I were going to have to remove my wig before I surrendered my colorful turban. The aide did not know.

I played solitaire for awhile. I had awakened early. I began to get drowsy. I didn't drink anything after midnight. My mouth was dry. Hanging out in the waiting area was boring. I worried about my hydration status and my potassium level. See-through liquids aren't very rich in potassium. If I'd used a "NO SALT" in my broth, I needn't have worried. I'll know better next time.

At last I was escorted to stretcher 28 in the preoperative receiving area. A woman came in and said, "I'm going to give you two OR caps and close the curtain so you can remove your wig and put these on. I'll put your wig with your belongings."

Then, the orderly transported me by stretcher to pre-anesthesia room 28. Two anesthesiology residents arrived and began their work. In no time I had an intravenous line in my right hand and midazolam on board and promises of fentanyl to come. The anesthesiology residents told me that I'd be awake when they wheeled me into the operating room.

I told the anesthesiologist in charge that I'd fallen asleep in the pre-anesthesia room the last time. She assured me that they wouldn't have let me go to sleep before I'd been taken into the operating room and attached to monitoring equipment. My memory of being in the operating room on my earlier journey had been completely erased, thanks to the medications that I'd been given.

While I was waiting, the door behind me opened and I heard a voice, "Hey, you!" I startled. It was Dr D. She told me that she'd called to find out if I was on the way. The person who answered the telephone didn't know what time I left. She'd told her that I was at the hospital. Since she had another woman waiting, she decided to switch the times. This was okay with me. I had to wait for my nephew!

I blurted out, "Hey, I get to see you in the OR this time." When I had had my previous surgery, I'd not seen her because I was "out to lunch" before they wheeled me into the operating room. Somehow I thought that I would be awake and participating in the procedure. The reality that I would be on the other side of the looking glass hadn't sunk it. Today was different. I knew that I would go to sleep.

I was still alert when the anesthesia residents came to bring me into the operating room. The operating room seemed to be very spacious. Dr. D was already present and all decked out in her personal protective attire (cap, gown, mask, eyewear, and gloves). I didn't recognize her.

The anesthesiologists instructed me to move onto the table, they attached the "wires" from the monitoring equipment to me, and they placed a mask over my face. One said, "We're giving you some oxygen to breathe. It won't put you to sleep."

Meanwhile the circulating nurse asked me, "How are you doing? Are you still cold?" I had about five blankets—several from the warmer—over me. I remember saying, "I'm okay now but I don't know what my doctor is going to say when I tell her that she can't take these blankets off." The nurse said, "I'm going to put some heavy leggings on so that I can put your legs in the stirrups. Is that okay?"

I remember that while she placed one on my left leg, the anesthesiologist was telling me that the oxygen wouldn't put me to sleep. I don't remember that she placed one on the right leg. The medications had kicked in.

The anesthesiologists gave me more medications in the IV tubing—cisatracurium and propofol and put a tube into my windpipe so that they could give me oxygen, nitrous oxide, and forane—the same gases that I'd received in January. Meanwhile the circulating nurse positioned me appropriately and made certain that I was kept warm. In contrast to the more complex surgery in January, today will be easier.

As soon as the anesthesiologists gave the go-ahead, Dr. D and her assistant made the initial small incision (~1/2-inch) to the left of my earlier incision. After measuring the pressure in my abdomen through a designated needle and inflating my abdomen with carbon dioxide gas, they inserted a trochar or instrument (~1/4-inch) through which she could place the laparoscope—the scope that would enable her to visualize the entire abdominal cavity. Except for a few small adhesions, everything looked normal! Next they made two small incisions and inserted two more trochars. They then obtained biopsies of small adhesions because no suspicious lesions were seen. At this time they learned that I'd been randomized to receive the clinical trial therapy. They placed a Tenckhoff catheter and secured it with a purse string suture. The instruments were removed and the incisions were sutured. Marcaine (a local anesthetic) was injected into these sites to prevent pain, and steristrips (little sterile tapes) were applied. Then the anesthesiology residents removed the tube from my windpipe.

The next thing that I remember after the nurse started to put leggings on is the anesthesia resident calling my name, "Theresa, hold your arms up in the air. Try to lift your head and shoulders." Most people call me Terry. It took me a minute to realize that they were talking to me.

I tried to hold my head and shoulders up but I couldn't for too long. As I did, I surveyed the room, looking in one direction and then the other. I thought, "Where is Dr. D? Where is she? Where is Dr. D? This is not good! Where is she?" Every time I lifted my head, I silently asked myself, "Where is L?" Later, she told me, "I was there at the time!" I have no doubt that she was there. I just didn't see her.

I heard the anesthesiology residents tell the anesthesiologist whom I'd seen earlier, "We tried to reverse her. We already gave her neostigmine." She told them, "You can repeat neostigmine." They did as she told them and I was able to obey their commands.

> Their conversation confused me. Neostigmine is used to treat myasthenia gravis (a neuromuscular disease in which a substance that enables nerve impulses to travel from one nerve to the next nerve is affected. Why did I need this medication?
>
> A few days later I located a pharmacology book and read that they had most likely given me an intermediate nondepolarizing agent (an anesthetic or numbing agent that interferes with the ability of nerve impulses to travel from one nerve to the next). When anesthesia is no longer necessary, the effect of this numbing agent can be reversed with neostigmine. According to my medical record, they gave me cisatracurium. This agent is used to provide skeletal muscle relaxation during endotracheal intubation (insertion of a tube into the windpipe) and during laparoscopy (insertion of a probe into the abdomen). This type of anesthesia is crucial during laparoscopy so that a patient doesn't move about and interfere with the surgeon's precision. Some antibiotics increase the effect of this drug. I overheard the anesthesiology residents discussing the fact that they wouldn't be giving me any antibiotics during this procedure. In contrast, antibiotics are generally given prior to laparotomy (incision into the abdomen) to prevent infection.

With a few minutes of my regaining a sustained ability to lift and hold up my head and shoulders, the nurse was providing me with discharge instructions,

"You need to return tomorrow to nuclear medicine at 11:00 AM." At this moment I became aware that I was in the experimental group. I would be receiving radioactive Yttrium.

Then the anesthesiology residents instructed me, "Move onto the stretcher. We're going to take you to the recovery room now."

My stay in the recovery room was very brief. At first I felt some discomfort and thought that the catheter in my bladder was still in place. However, I quickly ruled that out. If the catheter wasn't removed, I wouldn't be able to meet an essential standard for discharge—pass water. I wasn't sure why I was sore.

The recovery room nurse told me that my nephew had arrived at the surgical center but he left for while and would return later. She wanted to remove the unglamorous OR hats, but I panicked and said, "No, I'm not going to sit here without anything on my bald head. My hair had started to grow back in but it was very white, very fine, and very scant. I thought that I looked like a bald eagle. If it had been my natural color, it would have resembled five-o'clock shadow! I was adamant. Only my family saw me without my wig.

The nurse brought me ginger ale and saltines. I drank the ginger ale eagerly. After one bite I wanted to pass on the saltines because my mouth was so dry. She was insistent, "You have to eat the crackers before I can discharge you. You can have as much to drink as you want but you have to eat. I can get you more ginger ale."

I thought, "Man, these people are really tough." As a nurse I knew that I must be able to eat, drink and pass water before I could go home. I just wasn't as eager to eat as I thought that I would be after sixteen hours without fluid and nearly three days without solid food.

Suddenly my hand started to swell before my eyes. I called out to the nurse, "My hand is swelling!"

She looked at it and said, "It's not infiltrated. I'm going to get you up to the bathroom now. If you void (pass water), I won't have to restart it." I was willing to try. I was good at voiding.

As she helped me to the bathroom, I commented, "I can always use the facilities." I noticed blood back flowing up into the tubing. It hadn't infiltrated.

After a successful journey to the facilities, she removed the IV. She returned my worldly possessions and closed the curtains so that I could get dressed. She went out to find my nephew. She returned with him and with a wheelchair.

We made our departure. My nephew works for the Alarm Company that installed the security system in the surgical center. As my nephew pushed me in a wheelchair through the main lobby, he pointed out video cameras that he'd installed.

When we got outside I waited for him near the drive-through outside while he went for his van. I wasn't ready for a marathon but I was on my way home. I would be back the next day.

Being accepted into the clinical trial confirmed for the time being that I was in remission. My GYN oncology surgeon had taken a second look and didn't find any evidence of recurrent disease. If I hadn't been randomly assigned to the experimental condition, I didn't think that I would have been upset.

The following day July 2nd I arrived at the Nuclear Medicine Department. As Dee escorted me to the procedure room, she asked, "How are you doing?"

I commented, "I'm OK. Don't ever cross over. It's no fun."

She replied, "It's too late."

I looked puzzled.

She continued, "I already have. I had the same thing that you have?" She confirmed that she'd had ovarian cancer and she'd had radioimmune therapy.

I thought, "Wow! She really knows what I'm going through."

She removed the bulky dressing that my surgeon had used to cover the Tenckhoff catheter. As she hung a bag of normal saline and tubing on an IV pole and connected it to the catheter, she explained the procedure.

Following the infusion of 750 ml of normal saline (3 pints of salt solution), Dr F injected a radioactive imaging tracer into my abdomen. Then the staff encouraged me to roll from side to side and to walk for fifteen minutes. The intent was to disperse the solution and to verify that the solution was flowing throughout all four quadrants of my abdomen.

Images of my abdomen were taken and indicated that fluid wasn't flowing freely into some areas. I was encouraged to get up and walk and exercise for another thirty minutes. A second set of images yielded the information that the nuclear medicine physician was seeking. All areas of my abdomen were getting a fair share of the fluid. If this had not occurred, I'd not be able to receive this treatment.

After Dr. F administered Yttrium 90 HMFG1 antibody, another 300 ml of normal saline was infused into my belly. The surgical resident removed the Tenckhoff catheter. Now I needed to lie quietly until the opening created by laparoscopy closed over.

I knew that this normally occurred spontaneously in a short period of time. I'd cared for several children who had breathing tubes and feeding tubes at Children's Rehabilitation Center. If a tube was dislodged and another tube wasn't inserted promptly, the opening would shrink and a smaller tube might be needed. If too much time passed, reinserting another tube would be more complex.

Dee was concerned that I might be hungry. She gave ginger ale and wheat crackers.

A half-hour later my clothing felt wet. I called out, "Dee, I'm leaking a lot." She called the resident. He placed one suture at the site.

Fortunately I'd brought a change of clothing with me and was able to remove my very wet radioactive clothing. The radiation hazard team was called. They surveyed the area and identified "hot" supplies that needed to be isolated until the radioactivity potential deteriorated. Radioactive substances have what is called a half-life. During each half-life period, the radioactivity of a substance diminishes by half. This meant that they could predict when the "hot" supplies were no longer "potentially hazardous." This knowledge enables the creation of a safe environment so health care workers aren't unnecessarily exposed to excessive radiation. The only difference it made to me was that I didn't want to expose my family to radioactivity unnecessarily. The children were on vacation and wouldn't go near my "hot" clothing during Hide and Seek! They had already assured me that I would not be radioactive.

I had a small amount of additional leakage. The surgical resident placed two more sutures at the site. My clothing was slightly damp but I didn't have another set of clothing to change into. I was given detailed instructions for handling my belongings and I followed them meticulously. If I hadn't been a nurse who understood the importance of these instructions, they would've seized my clothing. I would've had to call my family and have them bring in more clothing.

I'd planned to stop at the snack area before I left for home, but my instructions were, "We don't want you to stop at the snack bar or sit anywhere else in the hospital." They gave me waterproof pads to protect the car seat from radiation.

Apparently my belly doesn't welcome a lot of fluid. If I've to have any more procedures that involve filling the belly with fluid, perhaps I should attach a 'pour at your own risk' sign to it.

For the most part the worst was over. I still had a marathon of health visits to undertake in the next few months but thus far I'd made a remarkable recovery. I was happy and thankful to be on the mend. My family and friends were happy for me.

12

Watching and Waiting.

Andrea set up a schedule of visits over the next six months. Checks were planned weekly for six weeks and then at 8 weeks, 3 months and 6 months later. The routine was the same: sign in at the desk, ask for a specimen container, fill the container, bring it to the laboratory, and have blood drawn, get weighed, have a blood pressure check, and complete a quality of life form. Then, after a brief interview and physical examination, I was on my way home.

The visits during the first eight weeks of the clinical trial coincided with summer vacations. The tedious routine was enlivened by the diversity of players on the team who saw me on a week-to-week basis. Having a cluster of caring, compassionate and competent physicians, nurses, and laboratory technicians transformed what might've been a real drag into an acceptable experience.

My first visit was with Dr D on July 9th. We talked about our encounter in preanesthesia room 28. My remembering absolutely nothing about my previous sojourn in the operating room triggered this conversation. I remarked, "I saw you before I went into the OR this time."

She replied, "You saw me in the OR."

I denied it, "No, I didn't!"

She persisted, "Yes you did. You saw me when you came in and you saw me before you left."

At first I didn't remember anything that she described. After my previous surgery, my brother and I were discussing our mutual experiences. He'd said, "It's kind of scary to think that they can give you something and you've no idea what happened." I nodded in agreement.

Of course, I'd wanted to be part of the action in OR 29 and not the object of the action. I was a little more amenable to being an object of the action in OR 28. Nonetheless, being on the other side of the looking glass wasn't where I wanted to be.

I recalled that I did see Dr D when they brought me in. She was all decked out in her personal protective equipment—OR attire. I didn't recognize her. I don't remember seeing her before I left the OR. I recollect looking for her to save me from the anesthesiology residents who were yelling at me to lift up my head and shoulders and try to hold them up for as long as I could. Being under anesthesia has funny effects as well as obvious benefits.

In spite of the fact that Dr. D knew that the anesthesiologists fulfilled their mission by making certain that I was tranquil, she was convinced that I'd seen her in the operating room. I'd been looking but I didn't see. I included the following note in my thank you letter to her after my surgery.

A Philosophical Anecdote

(right up there with)

"Why did the man who lost his keys in the darkness of the night look for his keys under the street light?"

If a sublimazed woman (who shall remain nameless to protect the guilty) looks without her glasses across the room at her *downtown surgeon* who is all decked out in her finest personal protective equipment and does not recognize her *downtown surgeon*, does the sublimazed woman actually see her *downtown surgeon*?

During the visit Dr. D had also asked me, "Are you happy that you received radioimmune therapy?"

I'd not really thought about this. I'd expected that I'd most likely be assigned to the control group. As I began to reflect on what having radioimmune therapy meant to me personally, it could represent added security. I responded, "Yes!"

After the late news on July 12th I had a nosebleed—my first nosebleed ever. My nose had been stuffy. I thought that I "blew too hard." Then I saw the blood. On a scale of 1–10 with 10 being the worst, I rated it a 10 plus.

The following week both Dr. D and Dr. S were on vacation. My appointment was with Dr P on July 15th at MGH. As I came off Sorrow Drive, traffic was moving very slowly. The sun was shining brightly. For the first time I noticed that fine hair was growing on my arms.

Things were going well. I mentioned my nosebleed. He said, "When we get your lab results, we'll take another look at your platelet count.

An assistant prepared to draw my blood. She was relatively inexperienced and her first two attempts were unsuccessful. She tried to persuade me to go to the main hospital laboratory where Gloria the world's best phlebotomist worked. I advised her that in my clinical practice I had a "three strikes and you are out" policy to protect the kids against the inexperienced. I suggested that she try the vein where "everybody who's anybody in the laboratory world" is able to draw my blood.

She reluctantly agreed to try this vein on the condition that I'd go to the laboratory if she was unsuccessful. I told her that I was hesitant to agree because her second attempt was kind of laid back and probably shouldn't count. She made one more try and she succeeded. Not only did she receive a boost in her confidence level but also I didn't have to go to the main hospital laboratory and wait for who knows how long!

Andrea gave me a supply of mail-out phlebotomy kits to bring back with me to the Cancer Center. I was certainly willing to bring a kit with me each week but I'd have enjoyed more fun presents.

The following week I met with Dr. S on July 22nd. I mentioned the nosebleeds. I'd had two more on the 20th. They were a 5 and a 1 on a scale of 1 to 10. They were less severe. He was not that concerned.

Dr. S was pleased to see how well I was doing. He said that he would look into alternating visits with Ricky the nurse practitioner. The principal investigator reviewed Ricky's credentials. Ricky had worked for the National Cancer Institute prior to coming to the Cancer Center. She passed muster.

While I was waiting in the lobby to be seen on July 30th, I observed a toddler running about. I commented to the woman sitting next to me, "Don't you wish you had bottled up some of your energy when you were his age so that you could have it now?"

She laughed. She shared some of her story. Although she didn't tell me what specific cancer she had, she told me that she would be on chemotherapy for the rest of her life. We discussed how we'd talked about our illness with children in our families.

I told her of my niece's response to learning that my hair would fall out but that it would grow back in again. She had responded, "That's stupid." My niece didn't like me to remove my wig. My scalp was sensitive to the turbans so I didn't wear them—even during the winter months. The woman told me that she didn't cover her head at home. Children in her family seemed okay with this.

Ricky saw me today for the first time since I completed chemotherapy. She was surprised and pleased to see how well I was doing. She was glad to hear that I'd had no nosebleeds since the 23rd. We discussed the study. The follow-up was intense.

My niece spent the day with me on August 5th. As soon as I got home, I usually took my wig off right away. I never wore the turban around the house because it hurt my scalp. In the past my niece was upset if I took my wig off. She'd say, "You look like a man." Trying to explain to her that not having hair on my head didn't make a person a man didn't work.

Today she was a lot more playful with my wig and my turbans. She enjoyed trying them on and looking at herself in the mirror. She wore the turban sideways. Her style was a lot more attractive. She was upset when I took her picture.

When I saw Dr D on August 6th, today, she was very interested in my continued peripheral neuritis and wanted to know if I thought that it was related to the radioimmune therapy. I didn't think that it was. My symptoms didn't get any worse but they didn't get any better either. I mentioned that I'd not had any nosebleeds since July 23rd.

I saw Ricky again on August 15th. I had more nosebleeds but none were serious. I think that I was more proficient with my first aid response. After applying local pressure, I usually applied a scant amount of Vaseline to my nostrils—a recommended treatment of nosebleeds. My platelets continued to be within normal limits.

I set out to meet Irma and Sister B for lunch on August 24th. I was the first to arrive. Irma joined me and we sat outside and chatted while we waited for Sister B. We waited and waited. Sister B didn't show up. Finally we decided that we should have our lunch.

We tried to explain why Sister B forgot to show up. We laughed as we conjured up reasons why she forgot us. Being forgetful wasn't unusual for her. We kept coming back to her sense of urgency that we get together much sooner than usual.

Later Irma called the convent and learned that Sister B had a relapse. She'd entered the order's nursing care facility and was dying. She passed away before I was able to visit her.

When I saw Dr D on August 27th, she wanted to know more about the nosebleeds. I'd sent her a graph that showed that they were subsiding.

They may've been related to residual lesions in my nose. Chemotherapy can irritate the mucous lining of the digestive and respiratory systems and cause lesions. Mouth sores are common. My nose had been crusty. When the nasal hairs started to grow back, the nosebleeds started. Neither Dr. D nor I thought that they were related to radioimmune therapy. I didn't know it yet but I'd had my last nosebleed.

During this visit Dr. D asked, "Are you going to let us see your hair today?"

Reluctantly I removed my wig.

She exclaimed, "You look cute. You have enough hair. You don't need the wig."

My hair was very white, very short, and very fine. I didn't think that I looked cute. I responded, "Oh, I look awful."

She continued, "You have a nice looking head. Believe me, I know. I have seen a lot of bald women. You could get a little color."

I read that hair dye shouldn't be used. I asked, "Is it okay? I thought that I couldn't."

Dr. D asked Gail, "Have you heard anything about not using color?"

Gail said, "No. Get a little color and wear some dangling ear rings."

As soon as I left the Cancer Center, I headed to my hairdresser's salon. She applied color to my hair and styled my wig. Dr. D wanted me to lose the wig, but I wasn't brave enough to go without it yet.

Initially I worked around the yard without it. The neighbor's dog didn't recognize me and barked incessantly. This was very annoying.

After a few weeks I went to the corner drug store or shopping without it. It was almost Halloween before I went to work without the wig. Not looking vulnerable in the workplace was important to me.

Dr S had an emergency at the hospital on September 23rd and was unable to get back to the Cancer Center for my appointment. Ricky covered for him. She commented, "This study is really keeping you busy. Isn't it?"

Sighing with relief, I responded, "I am finally on a three month schedule. You can't imagine what a relief it is." I continued to do very well.

One year ago today October 5th I had the symptom that launched the train that propelled me on this journey. I didn't remember that this was the anniversary. It promised to be a good day. I went to the VA Hospital where I have been doing volunteer work for over 40 years. We sponsor a monthly Bingo and refreshments. The recreational therapists were anxious to see me. "You have to talk to Kevin. He's having a tough time."

When Kevin saw me, he was relieved. He was distraught. He revealed that he had kidney cancer and would be having surgery at MGH in a few weeks. I was able to explain everything that he would experience from the moment he arrived for his preoperative assessment, through his surgical admission and hospital stay, and his return home. As I spoke I could see his tension diffuse and relaxation move in. I gave him my numbers—home phone, cell phone, beeper—and instructions to "call me anytime". He called me after his surgery to tell me that everything went exactly as I'd said it would. His surgeon told him, "We got it all." Kevin didn't need chemotherapy or radiation. I see him at least once a month and he keeps me updated on his progress.

Nearly two years after my primary care physician suggested a sigmoidoscopy, I finally had a colonoscopy on November 22nd. The prep was similar to but not as intense as the prep for the laparoscopy. Iron, aspirin, and coumadin aren't allowed for one week before the procedure. After a light breakfast the day before, only "see through" fluids, any gelatin except red, and juice without pulp are on the menu.

The instructions include Fleet Phosphosoda in the evening and in the morning and tons of juice or water. I decided to include favored oral electrolyte solution as part of my fluids and to drink them more gradually. This worked for me. I retained all fluids. I wasn't worried about a low potassium level. The good news was that I didn't have to take any enemas!

When I signed in, I learned that Dr. E would be doing the procedure rather than Dr. W. I didn't know either physician so it didn't matter to me. I thought that it was strange that they didn't tell me about the change ahead of time.

My sister-in-law dropped me off on her way to her own physician's office. The admitting clerk wanted to know why I was having a colonoscopy rather than a sigmoidoscopy. I said "The tumor had been very near my gut—too close for comfort." I wondered, "Who would volunteer for this if it wasn't necessary?" She needed to obtain an explanation that would satisfy the third party payers.

A long wait was ahead. I brought journals to read. The usual waiting area was being renovated and the temporary area was crowded. A woman came to the door behind me and called her husband. As they walked down the corridor together, I over heard her say, "Oh, this was worse than the colonoscopy!" I resisted my desire to run after her and say, "What test did you have?" Whatever procedure she had wouldn't make my wish list.

After awhile a nurse called me and escorted me to the change area. Once again, I changed into the unflattering hospital gown and robe and returned to a waiting area.

The nurse returned for me and led me into the procedure room. She explained what she'd be doing and started an intravenous line. She gave me meperidine (for pain relief) and midazolam (for sedation) through the IV line.

Dr. E explained the procedure. Colonoscopy is the insertion of an endo-scope—a long flexible tube—through the anus and advancement of the long flexible tube the entire length of the large intestine or colon to its junction with the small intestine. During the procedure they inflate the bowel with a gas (carbon dioxide). If the examiner sees polyps, the polyps are snared, cauterized, and retrieved. Then they are packaged and sent to the pathologist for examination.

They told me to pass gas during the procedure. I passed a lot of gas. I was doing fairly well until the end. At this point, I tensed up and told them, "I can't do this anymore." I sounded like a woman in labor who had reached the point of no return but claims, "I can't do this anymore." Although I didn't know it, the end was in sight for me.

The nurse asked, "Should we give her something else?"

Dr. E said, "It won't help." Imminently he was done. What he apparently meant was that since he was almost done, the medication wouldn't work in time to ease any discomfort. I didn't care what he meant. He was done!

They took me to the recovery room. While I was there, Dr E showed me pictures that he had taken and told me that I had a one cm. (less than ½ inch) sessile polyp but it was benign. He said, "You need to come back every 3–5 years." He wrote, "Repeat in three years."

I saw Dr. D on December 17th. It has been almost six months since radioimmune therapy. She was pleased with my progress. I noticed that she was preparing to test my stool for blood. I told her, "I finally got enough courage to have the colonoscopy that I had put off earlier. Dr. E said that it was benign. My primary care physician hadn't sent me an official pathology report yet." Dr. D printed a copy of the report for my record and a copy for me. The report was good.

I said, "This is a relief. I don't need any more problems."

Thus far, I was doing well after radioimmune therapy. I didn't seem to have any adverse affects from the treatment. The nosebleeds were apparently the sequelae of the effects of chemotherapy on nasal mucous membranes. The peripheral neuritis was also an effect of chemotherapy. I was disenchanted by the apparent slow return of my hair. I was expecting to wake up on or about the first of July with a full head of hair. Obviously I didn't. When my hair returned, it was very fine and thin, not like my thick hair before chemotherapy.

None of my laboratory results or symptoms seemed to be affected adversely by radioimmune therapy. I had a bit of an increase in the CA 125 that Dr. P said is normal. My platelets had varied within normal limits after both chemotherapy and radioimmune therapy. My white blood cell count had decreased to the low normal range after chemotherapy and had started to increase prior to the laparoscopy. They continued to rise steadily. The trend toward decreasing red blood cell count after chemotherapy, indicating anemia, had reversed itself preoperatively and was within the low normal range by July 31st. Two liver function tests fluctuated in the slightly elevated range after chemotherapy. The results after radioimmune therapy were comparable. When Laura called me with my test results, she consistently reported that "the laboratory tests looked good" and they did. I looked good. I felt great.

It was almost one year since my original surgery and nearly six months since the second look and confirmation of my being in full remission. I was now on an every three-month check and probably would be for another two and one-half years. Then I could be on an every six-month check until the end of the clinical study.

On February 1, 2003 our auxiliary had planned bingo and refreshments at the Edith Nourse Rogers Veterans Administration Medical Center. In the 1960s ten to twelve women used to go to the hospital on the first Friday evening of the month for bingo and refreshments. About 125–150 patients would come to the recreation hall where we held the bingo. As the years passed, our members got older and fewer women were able to go to the hospital. Some women were unable to drive at night. We started to schedule our activities on the first Saturday afternoon of the month. About 36–48 patients come to bingo.

As I headed toward the hospital, I listened to the radio. People were being warned not to approach the debris. The announcer was emphasizing that the debris could be toxic and no one should try to handle it. They should contact the local authorities. It sounded like something out of a science fiction movie.

After several minutes I became aware that the announcer was describing the wreckage of the Columbia space shuttle that had disintegrated upon reentry into the earth's atmosphere. Initially I didn't understand what he was saying. Gradually I realized that the shuttle had exploded upon entry into the atmosphere and its debris had been scattered over several states. Seven brave astronauts had lost their lives.

Memories of the destruction of the Challenger on takeoff several years earlier flooded my mind. The look of horror on Marlene's face as she came out of room 201 at the Children's Rehabilitation Center and revealed what had transpired was a sobering moment. We'd been excited to learn that the first teacher to go into space would be aboard the Challenger.

Later Janice had something urgent to tell me. The staff thought that a nurse should be selected to go up in space. Some of the staff had thought that I should be the first nurse to go up in space. Janice wanted me to know that what had happened on the Challenger wasn't what they had in mind for me.

Our country was saddened by the loss of these astronauts. We prayed that this would never happen again. Now it did. We couldn't believe it.

I stopped to take on a passenger on my way to the VA. I asked, "Have you been listening to the radio?" She'd heard. We talked about the disaster as we drove to the hospital.

The men and women at the VA had been watching the news when we arrived. They'd served in the Armed Forces and knew what it was like to lose their comrades in battle. Today they were subdued during bingo and refreshments. I felt that we couldn't have been in a better place on a day like this. We were with our American heroes on a day that our country lost seven of its astronauts.

They had valued our being present to them during this time. Everyone expressed the importance of our presence as they left the recreation area to return to their nursing units.

A three months check-up had been scheduled with Ricky on March 25th. It had been nine months since radioimmune therapy. After a thorough examination, we discussed how well I was progressing.

My Fiftieth High School Class Reunion was held on May17th. We had a great turnout! My life's journey took me down a very different pathway than most of my classmates. Although I'd seen a few former classmates at the local hospital either as parents bringing new children into the world or as nurses, I didn't have contact with many. Some hadn't changed much. Others had. Everyone looked great. I always like going to reunions because I look younger than most of my classmates.

Some of the hilarity of the evening focused on an acquaintance who was sitting at our table. About five years earlier, Richard had had open-heart surgery. I didn't remember an announcement of his passing on at the 45th Reunion, but this rumor had somehow got out. He laughed about life underground and his return to life above ground.

Richard looked for his first love—a girl whom he'd invited for an ice cream soda at the local drug store soda fountain when they were in third grade. Although he'd politely asked for "Two straws please", his first love guzzled the whole soda down in a very long slurp and he never even got a little sip. His first love didn't attend the reunion. We enjoyed his tale of his first attempt at a romantic life.

When he learned that I was a nurse, he told me about his *Near Encounter with Death*. I told him about the *Views from the Other Side of the Looking Glass: My*

Journey with Ovarian Cancer and what it was like to be on the high speed express train. He also told me that he earned his Ph.D. in chemistry and is a toxicologist.

I commented, "An acquaintance of mine recently died from beta cell lymphoma. When I read her obituary I learned that she had been a machinist. I suspect that workplace exposure to toxic substances may have been a factor."

Richard responded, "Not 'may have been', was." Apparently I said, 'may have been' again. He repeated, "was a factor." He explained that his life's work focuses on identifying toxic substances that are related to cancer. He described how he employs nurses to review medical records for him in an effort to establish linkages between these substances and various cancers. He gave me the name of two work-related chemicals and known carcinogens that she would've been exposed to. I asked him to write them down as I'd never remember them.

The Fiftieth Anniversary Reunion Committee of the Class of 1953 did an outstanding job assembling a souvenir book that highlighted stories about our classmates. Ninety-three (28%) of the 367 graduates attended the reunion. Although 59 (16%) of the 367 graduates are deceased and couldn't attend, most of the remaining 215 (56%) didn't attend for unknown reasons. Sixty-six of those who attended and three who weren't able to attend shared their stories in writing while the remaining 27 shared their oral stories at the reunion.

In their stories some described spouses, children, and grandchildren as a source of "pride and joy"; others spoke of enduring friendships and widening their horizons—36% live out of state. Some spoke of unanticipated success in the wake of discouragement by some teachers—some were told to drop out and get a job. Others shared stories of expected success as a result of motivation by other teachers—being asked, "Have you considered college?" Many described their diverse career pathways—medicine, nursing, teaching, chemistry, engineering, law, broadcasting, industry, office management, and legal assistant. Others spoke of military service—West Point, Air Force, National Guard, Coast Guard, or defense work—building nuclear ships and patriot missiles.

As I reflected on the stories of my classmates from the class of 1953, I thought about Crista McAuliffe's words to the children of America as she prepared for her journey into space. She encouraged the children to REACH FOR THE STARS. If a person couldn't actually grasp the stars, one would still go further than if he or she reached for the ground. Those who reach for the ground have nowhere to fall if they don't meet their goal.

As I look back on the last fifty years I am awed at the progress that has been made during this time. Members of the Class of 1953 who reached for the stars played an important role in this progress. To build on our achievements, I encouraged the Class of 2003 to "Dare to dream—to believe in their ability to fulfill their dreams—to create wonderful stories that they can share with one another at their Fiftieth Reunion in 2053—to find a way to share their wonderful stories with the class of 2053 and give them hope to move on and to encourage the next generation.

A reunion is never complete without a group photo. Unlike our class photo that was taken outside in 1953, this photo was taken indoors. Getting all of us into a small room at King's Inn was quite a feat. When the group photo arrived in the mail, I opened it eagerly. I recognized my smiling classmates instantly but the photo didn't seem to capture the event as I remembered it. I stared at the photo for several minutes. There I was on the opposite side of the room. How did I get there? After a while I discovered that the photographer had developed a mirror image of the group. My classmates had unknowingly joined me on the other side of the looking glass. A few weeks later the photographer sent us another photo. This one captured the event as it happened.

My annual Bone Density Examination and Mammogram were scheduled on May 27th. My primary care physician thought that it would be easier for me if I had them both on the same day. When I went to patient registration, the receptionist gave me a booklet detailing their new privacy policies that were recently mandated by the Federal Government. She said, "The Bone Density is no longer being done in the Women's Health Center. Take the first right after Radiology then the next left. Wait in the waiting area."

I followed her directions and walked past Radiology and turned right. If I continued straight, I would've walked into Cardiac Rehab. I was familiar with this area because one of my students had a clinical experience with a nurse preceptor in this setting.

When I turned left, I saw a few chairs in a rather crowded corridor. This was the "waiting area". While I waited, I keep my face buried in my journals as much as I could. The corridor was near an entrance to the hospital from the parking lot. People were coming and going. Whenever I looked up, I saw the sign that warned, "**CAUTION: RADIATIVE MATERIALS**."

I had a hard time concentrating on my reading. I kept looking at that sign. I realized that I would be taken into this area for the Bone Density Examination. It's one thing to go into the area when you need to be treated. It is quite another when you have no need to go there.

A woman came by and asked me my name. I answered. She commented, "You are kind of early, aren't you."

I replied, "I followed the instructions for arrival. Patient Registration sent me right over."

Finally the technician who would do the Bone Density Exam called me. I following her past the sign on the door, "**CAUTION: RADIATIVE MATERIALS**" into a small room on the immediate left. The room was so small that the chair where the technician sat to program the computer was partway into the hall. The door didn't close. After she positioned me and programmed the computer, she left me for awhile and the machine did its stuff. I could hear her talking on the telephone. She was discussing an exchange of x-ray film envelopes. Apparently someone else was having the same tests as I was but in reverse order. She returned and repositioned me and the machine did some more of its stuff.

The lack of privacy was upsetting. My hips and knees were bent and positioned on a padded block in a room with the door wide open on the day that I received the new booklet detailing their new privacy policies that were recently mandated by the Federal Government. However, a bone density is as easy as it gets.

When the examination was completed, the technician asked me, "Is your mammogram being done in the Women's Health Center or in Radiology?"

I responded, "To the best of my knowledge, it is being done in the Women's Health Center! But I was told that the bone density would be done there and here I am."

She handed me a large x-ray film envelope that contained several dozen x-ray films and asked, "Please bring this to the Women's Health Center with you." She gave me directions via the long route to the Women's Health Center. I looked at the name on the large x-ray film envelope. It wasn't mine. As I rounded the last corner I saw the door to the other side of the section where I had just been open. Here the sign was more ominous: **CAUTION: RADIATION AREA—RADIO-ACTIVE MATERIALS—AUTHORIZED PERSONNEL ONLY.** The technician exited. The Women's Health Center was a few doors down.

When I arrived at the Women's Health Center, I gave them the large x-ray film envelope containing someone else's x-rays. After I completed a questionnaire, I was instructed to go to the change room, take off everything above the waist, and put on the traditional hospital gown and wait. The area was very small and poorly lit. Not exactly the spot where an avid reader could stretch out and forget where she is.

I gathered my belongings and went into the corridor and tried to read one of my journals. When the technician came, she said, "You could've left your belongings in there." She brought me into the room where the mammogram would be done. The room is cozy. The walls are rose colored. The lighting is subdued. She explained, "We have a new machine. I am going to have to take a lot more films today."

In the past four films were characteristic. Occasionally the technician took an extra film. In the past I have been called back because the radiologists didn't like what they saw or couldn't see on a film. Twice I was sent for ultrasounds. Once I was sent to a surgeon whose specialty is breast cancer. I always got good news. After giving me good news, the surgeon told me, "You made my day. Today I've had nothing but bad news for everyone else."

Today she took ten films. I think, "This is never going to end." Silently I decide, "Surely they didn't miss anything today!"

Well, the radiologists did find something that they couldn't see clearly. I was called back to radiology this time to the higher tech equipment and the more experienced technician. The lights were bright, the walls were bright, and the equipment was in sight. The technician emanated caring, compassion, and competence. I felt that I was in good hands. She carefully took a few films and went out to develop them. She came back and sensitively tried another position. She seemed to know what would work. She went out to show the films to the radiologist. When she came back, she said, "He liked these and said to tell you, 'see you next year'." This was a welcome relief.

I had a CT Scan on June 17th as a part of the SMART Study Protocol. It went smoothly. The only thing that I forgot about and was quickly reminded of was the warm sensation in the bladder after the technicians inject the contrast dye. I'm getting to be an "old pro" at this.

My follow-up a week later with Dr D went well. I told Gail that I'd had the CT Scan but I forgot to pick up the films and report. She accessed the report on the computer. When she returned to recheck my blood pressure, Gail said, "She said to tell you that the CT Scan is fine." After Dr. D examined me, I was on my way.

My second celebration of National Cancer Survivors Day was on June 29th. Now I know that survivorship is measured from the time of diagnosis. In my case my diagnosis was revealed on January 11, 2002—on the day of surgery. I spoke briefly with Dr. S. He commented, "You look good." I told him about my conversation with my former classmate (the toxicologist) and promised to send him the names of the chemicals that he had mentioned.

One year ago today August 27th, Dr D suggested that it was time to lose the wig. I had my hair colored but I was slow to shed the wig. When I saw Dr. D in June, she suggested that I needed a haircut. My hair was so thin and sparse that I thought that I would simply let it grow out. My plan was "to never have another haircut again!" It surprised me that so little hair could be so hot in the summer time. I finally decided that it was time to shed a little. I felt as if I was having my first haircut ever. I watched as they swept up my hair into the dustpan and wondered if I should save a lock. I still have a lock of hair from my first real haircut ever. I decided against it. For the first time ever I had my hair teased. It looked good on the first day. It didn't look so good the next day.

Another three months recall on September 23rd. Sign in, ask for a specimen container, collect a specimen, go to the laboratory for blood draw and see Ricky! She asked, "Why are you seeing me and not Dr. S. I explain, "Amanda is now booking my appointments and didn't follow the schedule that I had sent to

Andrea. I'll emphasize the importance of following the schedule and see how she does with it." She didn't notify me when she made this appointment. When I called to find out if my visit had been scheduled, it was too late to change it.

She asked, "Are you doing some research?"

I explain, "I'm still planning to do a meta-synthesis on women's experiences with GYN cancer. I got started on writing a book about my own experiences with ovarian cancer and I got on a roll."

She is interested in hearing this. A close family member has fallopian tube cancer. There is nothing on this cancer. I know that she is right because I've been doing a lot of reading lately and have done some searches.

My niece came over after school on October 14th because her grandmother was having a diagnostic examination. It was her mother's birthday. We were planning to visit her mother's grave after her grandmother returned home. Several years ago I read that people who work with children who lost their mothers to AIDS had children write messages to their deceased mothers, attach them to balloons and release the balloons on important days.

She was eighteen months old when her mother was killed in an auto accident just two weeks to the day before Princess Diana was so tragically killed. Her brother was nearly seven years old. I suggested that we attach messages to their mom and release them on her birthday. We have done this for several years.

I suggested that she might like to make some tags that we can attach to the balloons. She went to work. She made a picture and wrote a message on a tag for each member of the family. She drew a picture of a unicorn from herself, a picture of a cat playing with a mouse from me, and a picture of a cat eyeing a bird from her great-grandmother. She drew another cat playing with a ball of yarn for her grandmother, an eagle from her grandfather, and a lizard from her brother.

My niece has inherited her mother's artistic talent. She enjoyed hearing a story that I told her about her mother.

When your mother was seven, she liked to go to work with me in the summer. "While I was at a meeting, she folded colored paper into quarters and made greeting cards. The faculty loved them and bought them for five cents each. She usually earned a dollar when she came to work with me.

Gen asked, 'Don't you have any with mice? I love mice.'

She left and returned a few minutes later with a birthday card. She had drawn a picture of a mouse nibbling at a birthday cake.

Gen commented, 'You were hiding the best cards?'

She answered, 'No. You said that you wanted a card with a mouse. I drew this one for you!'"

Her grandmother called to say that she was on the way to the cemetery with the balloons. We headed to the cemetery to meet her. It was almost dark. I was worried that they might've locked the gates. They hadn't.

We attached our tags to the balloons. We had additional messages. Some were long. I did my best to write them in the dark. I believe that people in heaven are able to read messages that are scribbled in the dark.

One by one we released the balloons. Gentle breezes in the air sent the balloons in different directions. After we finished, we went out to eat. My niece told her grandmother the story about her mother that I'd shared with her.

Unfortunately my nephew wouldn't join us. Instead of going home after school as his grandmother had asked, he went to a friend's house. He'd been having a hard time dealing with his mother's death recently and didn't want to go to the cemetery. He'd come with us in the past. His grandmother took him there the next day.

Often when the family gets together we share our memories of events during their mother's childhood and her siblings' childhood. Although her sister and her brother may say, "Oh, no, not that story", they seem to enjoy hearing stories of their childhood. Hearing stories about their mother's childhood has taken on an important role in keeping their mother's memory alive.

My nephew wanted to be included in our memories. He said, "I have a story about me. One day my mother said, 'Come on. We need to go to Brooks Pharmacy to get your sister's medicine.' I thought, 'Wow, I've been to Brooksby Farm to pick apples several times and I never knew that they sold medicine.' When I got there I knew that we weren't going to be picking apples."

The fortieth reunion of our nursing class took place on November 1st. Although four men and thirty-three women graduated with us, two of the 37 graduates whose education had been interrupted were members of an earlier class. One member of our class had taken a leave of absence and didn't graduate for another year. Twenty of the 36 graduates who had entered the nursing program together attended the reunion. Three couldn't be located. Some couldn't attend because of distance. At least three of the graduates had earned a master's or higher degree in nursing. Two were widowed. Four of five classmates who were deceased had died from cancer. The fifth classmate died from complications after surgery.

Two of the twenty who'd attended had transient medical problems and were unable to work. Two were planning to retire. One graduate has been a model. The remaining graduates were still actively employed in nursing. They were employed in a variety of hospital-based and community-based settings.

Stories that were shared during the reunion included oral reminiscences of nursing in the early 1960s and the transformation of nursing to what it is today. Our educational pathway was very different from that of nursing students today. We remembered several patients who had been in the hospital while we were nursing students. We also recalled stories about the people who had played a role in our earlier development. I mentioned getting a get well card from a former evening supervisor. She'd written, "I don't know if you remember me or not but I was evening supervisor for the back of the house." In unison, everyone spoke, "Who could ever forget Mrs. A?"

Mary and Maureen, two clinical nursing faculty, who were always available for us on evenings provided much appreciated guidance and support to us as we struggled with the responsibilities of being in charge on evenings. During our sojourn at a hospital school of nursing, we were given much more responsibility than are current nursing students. Most of us realized that we couldn't have done it without Mary and Maureen.

As I reflected on my classmates' stories, important themes seemed to emerge. In many ways things were better then. We were closer to our patients. We weren't dependent on technology. We had to rely on our observations and interpretive skills. In other ways the situation is better now. Medical advances have enabled patients who didn't survive in the past to survive today and receive supportive care in the community. While it's good that people can go home sooner, it's unfortunate that people are being sent home too soon and care is being rationed.

I didn't get a sense that my classmates wanted to go back to the way things were. I did get a feeling that as health care becomes more technology oriented they didn't want to lose sight of the human touch that has been so important to us. Caring and compassion were very important and were the foundation of our nursing practice.

From my perspective substituting reliance on technology for clinical judgment compromises our effectiveness as nurses. While I was at Children's Rehabilitation Center, Julie told me this story. "While I was making rounds everything on the monitor looked fine. He was sleeping peacefully on his belly on the mat. I hated to disturb him but something told me to check. I turned him over and he was blue. The readout on the monitor still looked fine. I'm glad that I checked him." In spite of the fact that we had a State of the Art monitoring system, her use of clinical judgment and her early detection of a problem were crucial and had benefited the child.

We went to the VA Hospital on November 8th for our customary Bingo and refreshments. Kevin who had renal cancer and surgery was happy to tell me that his CT Scan was negative. This was great news. We rejoiced!

Although I know that follow-up is important I was getting tired of so many recall visits. I calculated the number of visits remaining after my next check-up as being between eight and twelve. I started the countdown. I thought that this would help.

Within a few days Amanda called me to tell me that she'd scheduled an appointment with Dr. D on December 23rd. She told me that the SMART Study was coming to a close. This wasn't surprising. I'd just received a letter that indicated that 220 women had received Radioactive Yttrium. The goal had been to enroll 420 women in the study. Approximately one-half of the women would be randomized to the experimental group (receive Radioactive Yttrium) and the remaining would be randomized to the control group (receive standard care). Their enrollment goal had been achieved.

My recall visit with Dr. D on December 23rd went well. We discussed follow-up now that the SMART Study would be coming to a close. Dr. D told me that I no longer needed check-ups every three months. She said, "On your way out today, make an appointment to see me in six months." Hearing this news was exhilarating!

In a way going back for check-ups is like waiting at the train terminal on stand-by. Only I hope that they won't find a seat for me on the train. I have no desire to get on the train—the high speed express train—the train that will take me where I don't want to go.

When I came in today, I anticipated waiting at the train terminal on stand-by for about 8–12 more times. When I left, I realized that I might only have to show up about 5–6 more times.

My fourth routine annual health examination with my current primary care physician was scheduled on January 16, 2004. She asked the typical questions and made notes. She commented "We had several cancellations because of the weather." It was very cold today. I didn't tell her that I was hoping that she would call and cancel. I knew that she did her residency at the Mayo Clinic in Rochester Minnesota. Last year she had told me about typical winter weather during her residency. She wasn't likely to cancel.

She took her time and listened very carefully to my breathing and heart sounds, assessed my nervous system status, and prescribed cholesterol screening. Later I would learn that my cholesterol level had risen.

I didn't do too well trying to walk on my heels. I attributed this transient diminished functioning to the cold weather.

She asked, "Are your [toes] painful?"

I think, "The peripheral neuritis in my feet and hands still plagues me. The bedcovers weigh heavily on my feet. The computer keyboard wrecks havoc with my hands. My overall health is excellent. Her greatest challenge since becoming my primary care physician has been managing the annoyances that beset us when our warranties run out. I don't want her to say the B word. I don't want another problem added to my problem list."

I respond, "Not much. It's hard to get shoes that fit."

She recommended a brand of shoes that is available in wide sizes.

My mother's annual eye examination was scheduled on January 21st. While sitting in the waiting room, I overheard an assistant call Maureen M into the exam area. The name was familiar. I had known Maureen M over 40 years ago. I looked up to see if I recognized her. I did. I wondered if I would've a chance to talk with her. While I was waiting with my mother for her eyes to dilate, Maureen was escorted to this area.

I said, "How are you?"

She exclaimed, "I know you from somewhere."

I replied, "Lynn Hospital." She'd been an operating room nurse for several years.

She asked, "What are you doing now?"

I answered, "I retired last spring."

She continued, "I did too. I had to. I was forced into it. I had [multiple] myeloma (a cancer that involves the bone marrow and a cell that produces antibodies). She went on to tell me her story. "I woke up. I caught my foot on the covers and broke my tibia and fibula (lower leg bones). They insisted that I must've fallen but I didn't! I caught it and it just crumbled. I no sooner finished rehab when somehow I twisted and broke three vertebrae (spinal bones). After surgery and their putting all kinds of pins and rods, I spent three months at Life Care. No one suspected myeloma.

Remember Sharon G. She saw me and said, 'You look awful. I'm taking you to the ER.' I remember being in the ER, but I don't remember anything for the next six months. I was diagnosed with advanced myeloma and they gave me three weeks. I don't remember a thing. I've been in remission for six years.

I mentioned to Maureen that a friend of a friend was being worked up for multiple myeloma. At time I didn't know what her diagnosis was but I expected to find out soon.

While others have already been on comparable journeys and have unique stories to tell, some are about to embark on expeditions into the unknown. Sharing our stories with those who're about to take off to unfamiliar places is one way of those of us who've been there can help ourselves as well as others.

When I went to the VA Hospital for our Bingo and refreshments on February 7th, Kevin approached me and said, "Guess what? I went to my regular doctor and he discovered that my prostate test was elevated." I've been doing some reading on prostate cancer and was able to share some of my knowledge with him. He knew a great deal about the disease. He told me that his uncle had had prostate cancer and didn't have surgery. He had died from another disease. He would be seeing a specialist and reviewing his options and he would keep me updated. In comparison to his earlier cancer experience, Kevin was a lot less anxious than he had been in November 2002 and was able to talk about taking things one day at a time.

On February 20th, another CT Scan was scheduled. Overall, the test was similar to my previous experiences. Unfortunately the barium drink resulted in more frequent trips to the facility than in the past. I was glad that I didn't have to drive into Boston.

Mary brought me into the pre-examination area, took a medical history, and inserted an IV catheter in my arm. Then she brought me into the procedure room with the more modern machine. It looks much less confining. The recessed ceiling has a pale blue background and soft white clouds and recessed lights. The setting is very relaxing. A relaxing environment was very helpful to me as I was distressed by the undesired barium aftermath.

Initially the procedure was going along as it had in the past. Then the technician told me that he would inject the iodinated contrast medium. Usually this material has stimulated a feeling of warmth in my bladder area. Today I felt a more generalized sensation of warmth over my body and in my mouth and was less aware of warmth in the bladder area than in the past. The unexpected sensations concern me and I planned to mention them to Dr. D when I see her in June. I forgot.

The fourth anniversary of the Ovarian Cancer Education Awareness Network (OCEAN) was celebrated on February 24th at MGH. I arrived early and visited the resource room before the event. When I went out into the lobby, Dr P was there. We chatted for a few minutes.

A woman who had ovarian cancer stage four spoke to me. She'd been referred to MGH by a community hospital in the Metro West area. She had her initial surgery in March 2002—just two months after I had my surgery.

When she saw her leading gynecologic oncologist he told her how they could approach her cancer. He said, "We won't give up on you. If this doesn't work, then we'll try this. If this doesn't work, then we'll try this. If this doesn't work, then we'll try this. If this doesn't work, then we'll try this…" She was aware from her initial visit that multiple approaches to her cancer were available and her future included the possibility of remission. I knew that she was in good hands because my surgeon would have trusted me to his care if she'd not been available to do my surgery.

I told her that I was excited to hear her story and see how well she was doing. I knew someone who had told me about her sister-in-law who had ovarian cancer stage 3 and had died several months ago. I also told her about Rita who was a survivor since 1968. Instantly she responded, "I need to hear stories like this!"

Hearing about women who have had good outcomes has been very important to me as well.

Two days later my primary care physician notified me that my CT Scan was normal on February 26th. Although this outcome was expected, this news was still welcome!

Our next Bingo for the veterans at the VA was March 6th. Kevin told me that he'd been scheduled for surgery in less than two weeks. He had a good understanding of what his before, during, and after surgery course would be like. I promised him that I'd keep him in my prayers. He would be in good hands.

13

Living with a Life Threatening Illness

As my early test results came in, I developed a pervasive sense of hopelessness and despair. My definition of the situation—cancer as a terminal illness—had emerged from my early experiences with patients who were in the late stages of varying types of cancer at a time when relatively ineffective treatment protocols were available. As I embarked on my current journey my definition of the situation has gradually changed. My outcome wasn't as dismal as I'd projected. The transition from despair to hope didn't occur magically. Each piece of evidence that my fate wasn't as bad as I'd imagined was weighed carefully much as a pharmacist would weigh a medicine that required precise dosing. I would ask myself, "Do I dare believe the evidence?"

In spite of my anxious filtering of each piece of information, I gradually became aware that my prognosis in comparison to others is very good. The evidence in my medical record supports this conclusion.

Early on, the evidence suggested the probability of some type of cancer. It just didn't reveal the type of cancer. The reports suggested a variety of options. My preference was "fibroid". After surgery the clinical reports confirmed early stage of ovarian cancer, but a very aggressive tumor—a far cry from my choice.

My response to the prescribed course of chemotherapy wasn't as bad as I had anticipated. I would've liked to trade some days in for better ones. For some reason I responded to the fifth round as if I'd had a double whammy. Yet the evidence on the medical record confirms that I had a reduced dose. The fact that I was in complete remission prior to entry into the SMART Clinical Trial—a criterion for entry—confirmed that my prognosis was good.

My response to Radioimmune Therapy was favorable. Although hematology values were still low when I entered the SMART Clinical Trial, abnormal clinical values had begun to be reversed prior to the laparoscopy and continued to rise after Radioimmune Therapy. The only exception was a slight rise in the CA 125—that according to Dr. P, was an expected response.

Things were going well when I received a call from Dr. P. He wanted to know if I would be willing to meet with a first year medical student during the spring 2003 semester. The medical student would be enrolled in a course that focused on learning what it was like for people who were *Living with a Life Threatening Illness* (LWLTI).

I wasn't sure how much a student would learn from me about *Living with a Life Threatening Illness*. I was doing very well but I wouldn't refuse a chance to educate a future physician about what patients need from their physicians. After I reviewed the course description, I called back to confirm my interest. I agreed to be a patient teacher and share what *Living with a Life Threatening Illness* (LWLTI) has been like for me. I met with the medical student weekly from mid March through late May.

Alex called me in February 2003. We set up a time and place to meet the following week. I fully intended to keep my appointment with her. A family crisis interfered with our plans to meet. My sister-in-law had a medical problem that had emerged gradually over the past year. She experienced shortness of breath that dated back to January 2002 when I'd had my initial surgery. Her physician's diagnosis was asthma. The prescribed asthmatic regimen was ineffective. In October she learned that she had an abnormal heart rhythm and underwent cardio version in an attempt to restore normal heart rhythm. In November she had a pericardiocentesis to remove excess fluid from the sac that surrounded and normally protected her heart. These therapeutic procedures provided temporary relief of her symptoms.

In February she was scheduled for pericardiostomy—a procedure that would relieve persistent excess fluid in the sac surrounding the heart. She was admitted to an in town teaching hospital early Monday morning. She expected to stay overnight and return home Tuesday morning. The children would stay with me from Sunday afternoon through Tuesday afternoon. I thought that I'd be able to meet Alex on Wednesday morning.

When the children came home from school on Monday, they were anxious to find out how their grandmother was doing. I promised them that I would call after supper. I anticipated that she'd be awake enough to say, "Hey, guys, I'm okay. Let me get a little more rest. I'll be home before you get home from school." After all, she was coming home the next day.

I didn't tell them that I was calling her. The first time that I called, the staff said, "Her nurse won't be able to come to the telephone for thirty minutes." I thought, "Damned staffing patterns." I called back an hour later. The nurse was still unavailable. I didn't like this. Supper hour was over—not that nurses ever get to go to supper. Something was very wrong and I didn't know yet what it was or how bad it was.

The children were asking, "Why can't we talk to her?" I'd not told them what was going on. Now I needed to give them a simple explanation. I explained, "She still has the tube in and she can't talk to us yet. I am trying to reach 'Grampy' so he can talk to us."

It was after ten o'clock before I got any information. They didn't tell me that she'd crashed and had been rescued but I knew. They did tell me that she had been sent to the Intensive Care Unit.

When I spoke with my brother, he was beside himself. "They're not telling me everything, anything. I asked them, 'How can she have low blood pressure? She is being treated for high blood pressure!'"

I'm not a cardiac nurse! It did occur to me that if they drained the extra fluid surrounding her heart that her heart would beat more efficiently. An adjustment in her antihypertensive medicines might be in order. I'd already prepared her to monitor her blood pressure closely when she came home. I wondered why her medical team didn't anticipate this response and put preventive measures in place.

Several days later my sister-in-law began to recover and was able to go home. In the meantime the children had a hard time understanding what was going on and why they couldn't talk to their grandmother.

After this delay my meeting with Alex was put on hold two more times. First she returned to the Great Northwest to visit her family during her school vacation. Then she called to tell me that her grandmother had died. She'd call me when she returned from the West Coast.

Alex and I finally got together about three weeks after her initial call. Needless to say, we didn't begin our dialogue about *Living with a Life Threatening Illness* right away. The process of living a life threatening illness doesn't go on in isolation. The rest of the world isn't out partying while we're going through our own turbulence. Life goes on and we have to deal with it.

Each week I met her at the University Medical School Bookstore. Being able to peruse the bookshelves kept me busy until she arrived. Usually we went for a walk around the Fenway. She generally wanted to walk a different path each week. On our first walk we passed by Charles McGilvray Park—a memorial park that honored veterans from Boston who had served our country. I told her that I had represented the State Disabled American Veterans Auxiliary at the Memorial Day Ceremonies during my sojourn as State Commander in 1998. The ceremony is impressive.

During our walks I described my experiences with this unwelcome intrusion in my life. She had many, many questions and I answered them as well as I was able to. At some point I started to develop an outline of my notes of my cumulative experiences. As I did, I began to review some of my notes that I had jotted down as I progressed through my illness, my early symptoms, diagnosis and treatment, and my responses to it.

I explained to her that I had frequently tended to be somewhat clinical when I kept notes about the various events that comprised my experience. I talked about how it seemed as if I was looking into a mirror at someone else who was going through this experience—someone else who'd found herself on the high speed express train. I'd read about other patients who said that having cancer was like being on a roller coaster. Not me! I was definitely on a train—a very, very fast train. It didn't slow down. It just kept going.

The train was always going so fast. Information was bombarding me like fly-ing bullets whizzing by. I needed it to slow down. Dr. D seemed to be okay with this. When I shut down, she eased back. When I opened up, she made sure that I got the amount of information that I could absorb. She didn't assume that I didn't need explanations because I was a nurse. When she explained the laparos-copy to me, she said, "I am going to talk to you as if you don't know anything." I nodded inwardly. This is what I tell my students to do when they are caring for physicians and nurses. This is what I needed now.

Alex, the first year medical student, realized that my confidence in Dr D's competence and her caring and compassionate approach was very important to me. I expressed my hope that she would meet with Dr. D, as this was a course expectation. If she did, she never told me. I had hoped that she would.

Alex wanted to know if there was a moment in time when I accepted my diag-nosis from an emotional perspective. I couldn't answer this question. Coming to terms with the reality of having cancer doesn't come magically. It takes time and effort. From an intellectual perspective, I knew that I had it. How could I not know? The facts struck me in the face like a ton of debris falling out of the sky from plane circling above, ridding itself of its toilet waste. From an emotional perspective I didn't fully integrate the experience into my life for a long, long time. I can't say how long this wavering back and forth took. It seemed to dimin-ish gradually over time. At some point I stopped thinking about not having can-cer and was able to say that I have it. I don't know when it happened. It just did.

I'd known almost from the beginning of my journey that the CA 125 wasn't very useful in the differential diagnosis of ovarian cancer. I'd not been able to confirm from my reading that the CA 125 was a useful indicator of the efficacy of treatment for ovarian cancer. In one of my e-mails to Dr. P, I made this com-ment about my results—"of course, I don't know what this means." When he responded, he wrote, "It means that you are in the best prognosis group." This is where I am—in the best prognosis group.

Again Alex asked, "Was there a specific time that you realized that you'd accepted your diagnosis emotionally?" I answered, "Not really. I could only absorb so much. Then I would back off. When I was ready, I was able to ask or look for more information."

My friend Mary affirmed my perception of denial's safeguarding role—tiding us over until we shore build up our resources again. As I reflected on Mary's affirmation, I recalled events surrounding the untimely death of my former colleague and friend Robin. Robin taught psychiatric nursing for several years at the Tri-City Hospital School of Nursing where I taught Nursing of Children. She was one of the few who appreciated my strong psychology background and we had many animated discussions. After each quarter the four faculty members who taught on the second level—Robin, Nancy, Cilla, and I—went out to lunch together. The Stone Zoo was our favorite spot after the spring quarter.

After Robin resigned to take another position, she came back to visit us on a Friday afternoon. I was very busy and spoke briefly with her. I joked with her for a few minutes. I didn't linger. Not long after her visit, we learned that Robin had died unexpectedly. If I had only known that I'd never see her again, I would've made time.

Although the Program Director had known the details of her death, she didn't share this information with faculty or students. Jayne who had taken Robin's place realized that something was amiss. She tried to compel us to deal with the reality of the circumstances of her death. Her efforts aroused my anger to incredible heights. Coming to grips with her death at this time was hard enough. Accepting the circumstances of her death at this time would've been too painful.

After some time had passed, I retrieved my copy of Shneidman, Farberow, and Litman's *The Psychology of Suicide* (Science House, 1970) and began to read it. Gradually I began to realize that my friend had taken her own life. My earlier denial had helped me during my initial intense response to her untimely demise. In time I was able to accept the reality of what had transpired. No specific moment of reality—just a wavering back and forth between denial and emerging acceptance and the eventual realization that she'd taken her own life.

This was how it was with me when I faced the possibility of cancer. Gradually I came to accept the reality that I had cancer. Moments of denial enabled me to control the volume of incoming information and quell my mounting anxiety.

The challenge that I face now is coming to terms with the possibility that I may have been cured. Dr. S's stated goal is CURE! Dr. D is optimistic. Dr. P tells me that I am in the best prognosis group. The judicious physician will proclaim cure after five years. The cautious physician may never proclaim cure.

Nonetheless, I am doing very well. The evidence on my medical record supports this. I realize that follow-up is crucial and I'll follow the standard guidelines. However, concerns about relapse are on the back burner. I am able to say "I may be cured" but I know that I won't be casual about my future.

Life takes us in many directions at the same time. Several years ago, while driving home from Maine, I saw a cluster of highway signs—9 East, 10 North, and 12 South. I stopped by the side of the road to take a picture of these markers. Some day, I thought, this cluster of signs could be the title of my autobiography!

Often we do not know where we are going because we are going in so many directions at once. Then cancer shows up. We are suddenly propelled in a direction that we don't want to go. But we must go where the speeding train takes us. To go there is to have the opportunity to transform devastation into hope. My experience with cancer is as if I swerved off the highway but I've been able to get my car back on the road and I'm continuing my journey. I'm back on the highway traveling in many directions but I'm looking forward to where life will take me.

14

Sorting out Souvenirs

Before setting out on a journey, most of us gather up inviting brochures that showcase places to see. We go on the Internet to choose a time to go, a place to stay, and a time to come home. We get to choose where we're going, whom we're going with, how we're going to get there, and what we will do. While we're on our journey, we take photos and pick up souvenirs from the places that we visit to bring back to our friends and family.

Not too long ago I rode on a train to New York City. The ride was leisurely. As the train slowed at the bend before Kingston station, I saw the ram that used to nibble grass near the side of the back road that I traveled on my way to the University of Rhode Island. As the train continued, a grand view of the University Campus that I'd never seen before came into view.

The train stops at Kingston station. One of my classmates from the University discovered a postcard picture of Kingston station while she was in Germany with her husband when he was on sabbatical. She sent it to me with a note: "Imagine having to go halfway around the world to get a postcard picture of Kingston station."

Not having to worry about traffic on the interstate on my way to New York City had been relaxing. In stark contrast, during my journey with ovarian cancer, the train was usually traveling at breakneck speed. Unwelcome questions bombarded me. How'd I get on this train? Where's it headed? What's happening? How am I going to get off? While I was thinking about everything that was happening so fast, I had to struggle to keep up. I couldn't relax and enjoy the scenery.

While I was on my journey I collected an assortment of books and journal articles about diagnosis and treatment of cancer, information about current research, available resources, useful Internet sites, and books by other people who'd lived through cancer experiences. From time to time I wade through my assorted souvenirs and try to make sense of my journey. One of my favorite souvenirs is a book by Suzanne Strempek Shea.

In her book *Songs from a Lead-lined Room: Notes—High and Low—From my Journey through Breast Cancer and Radiation*, Suzanne Strempek Shea tells a story about a bird who'd become trapped on the fourth floor of the tower at the Quabbin reservoir. I accepted an invitation to attend a class at Bayside College where Suzanne had agreed to read. Students who'd read her book found this passage to be meaningful. They'd asked her to read this passage.

After listening to her readings, I purchased a copy of her book from a local bookstore. The first time that I read about the bird flying against the window and being rescued by Suzanne, I perceived a sense of caring and compassion. She knows that she has to free the bird from its imprisonment. When the bird slips out of her grasp, Suzanne tries again. She cautiously wraps her scarf around the bird. She delicately carries the bird outside, removes the scarf that envelops it, and sets the bird free. The little creature awkwardly flies away. Suzanne watches for a few minutes and then continues on her journey.

A year later, I return to her story. As I reflect on the story of the little bird, I wonder, "How did the little bird get trapped in the tower? Why did the bird get into this predicament? How did I get into this predicament? Why did I get ovarian cancer? Will I be set free?" I don't know.

The answer to how I got ovarian cancer isn't simple. The diagnostic work-up indicated that I could have cancer of the lining of the womb or cancer in the area surrounding the womb. Although the radiology report favored a fibroid, my ovaries couldn't be seen. Ovarian cancer wasn't ruled out. As I perused the literature, I began to realize that I had several risk factors associated with both endometrial and ovarian cancer: having early onset of menses, having never been pregnant, being obese, having late cessation of menses, and being postmenopausal.

I favored the diagnosis of fibroids but I knew that the tumor was growing and not shrinking as a fibroid would at my age. My preference wasn't an informed choice. I also knew that atypical uterine bleeding is usually the first sign of endometrial cancer. I'd suspected that dietary attempts to reduce total cholesterol may have interfered with estrogen production and triggered bleeding and short cycle premenstrual-like symptoms. The initial symptoms prompted me to contact my primary health care provider immediately. As a result my cancer was found in an early stage and my prognosis is much better than it is for most women who are diagnosed with ovarian cancer.

As my journey continued, other questions perplex me: "Could I have prevented this?" "Is ovarian cancer preventable?" "How likely is it that ovarian cancer could be found in its early stages?" "Why was ovarian cancer in my case found in an early stage before it spread to nearby tissues?"

Cancer prevention involves reducing associated modifiable risk factors. No guarantees are made. Non-specific cancer prevention guidelines have been described in the literature. Certain guidelines address healthy lifestyle behaviors that could reduce the risk of morbidity (illness) and mortality (death). For example, protection from exposure to the sun and artificial sunlight is recommended to prevent skin cancer—the most common malignancy. Periodic examination of the skin is recommended to promote early detection and treatment. Most often the persons who have skin cancers are the ones who discover them. A friend recently had surgery for skin cancer on his face. He knows that he has to be careful about exposure to the sun. He keeps me posted on his progress. He is doing well.

Although lung cancer is the second most common cancer, it is the number one cause of death from cancer in men and women. Smoking is the leading cause of lung cancer and smoking increases susceptibility to lung cancer from other causes. Smoking increases the risk of cervical cancer, heart disease, and other diseases. Smoking abstinence is strongly recommended. In 2003 Gritz and colleagues urged smoking cessation in cancer patients: *never too late to quit*. They reported that nearly 31% of deaths from cancer are related to tobacco use and that smoking is associated with reduced cancer treatment effects and increased harmful effects of cancer treatment.

In mid-October 2003, I learned that a classmate from my first nursing program had died from cancer in June. I heard the announcement at the annual alumni meeting. I gasp. I couldn't have heard right. This must be a mistake. I knew that it was Liz but I had to check it out. I sought out the person who made the announcement to ask, "Is she the one who was in our class?" She was. Almost instantly, I knew that it was lung cancer. She was a smoker.

I've never smoked, but I've been exposed to an abundance of second-hand smoke in my lifetime. This is disconcerting. Institutions and organizations that forbid indoor smoking inside allow smokers to congregate at their entrances. People who enter and leave the buildings are exposed to second-hand smoke. Acquaintances who have had other cancers have not quit smoking. Everyday I see smokers congregating at the entrances of healthcare facilities and schools. I want to design a bumper sticker: **Enjoy breathing? Quit smoking!**

Breast cancer is the most common cancer in women. Breast cancer affects 1 in 8 women. One of my classmates from nursing school has already died as a result of having breast cancer. Women who have early menarche, late first pregnancy, or late menopause are at increased risk. Obese postmenopausal women are at increased risk. Women whose parents, siblings, or children and women who have the BRCA 1 or BRCA 2 gene are at greater risk of developing breast cancer.

Obesity is a risk factor in cardiovascular disease, diabetes mellitus type II, and some cancers, including ovarian cancer and breast cancer. If we reverse the trend toward increasing incidence of obesity, we can improve the overall health of the nation and modify the risk of <u>some</u> ovarian and breast cancers. The American Institute for Cancer Research and the American Cancer Society advocate a diet that includes fruits and vegetables and other foods that are derived from plants rather than animals. Physical activity to moderate weight is recommended. Obesity was my only modifiable risk factor. Previous attempts at weight loss had not been successful.

Several years ago a fellow student in the nursing doctoral program at the University of Rhode Island had asked me to complete a questionnaire. The questionnaire would be used in research conducted under the auspices of the Cancer Prevention Consortium at the university. They planned to study what people were doing to reduce fat in their diet.

At the time I was making an effort to cut back on sweets, but I wasn't doing much to reduce fat in my diet. I did a few things. I removed as much visible fat as I could. I bought the hamburger with the lowest percent of fat. I drank low fat milk for a while. I even used margarine instead of butter to reduce my cholesterol intake.

After I graduated, teaching nursing at a college in the area, continuing to volunteer in a variety of activities, and enjoying a variety of activities with friends and family kept me busy. It was tempting to stop at the neighborhood seafood take-out for a combination plate—a delicious meal that was loaded with fat! The busier I got, the more frequently I stopped at the local seafood take-out. What started out as a halfhearted attempt to cut back on fat was soon replaced by overwhelming effort to the contrary.

During a routine health care check-up, I learned that my cholesterol had taken a turn in the wrong direction. This wasn't good news. My risk for heart disease was increasing. I set out to reverse this trend. I was seriously overweight, but I didn't concentrate on calories. My focus was on maintaining a well balanced diet that incorporated elements of a low fat/cholesterol, low salt, and moderate carbohydrate diet. My objective was to lower my cholesterol level. I also hoped to prevent hypertension and diabetes mellitus.

I made serious changes in my diet and began to lose weight. My intent was to cut back on my stops at the neighborhood seafood take-out. I stopped altogether and substituted lobster rolls for fried foods. I made several other changes as well. I lost about two pounds a month—a weight loss well within the Guidelines of the National Institute of Health published in Obesity: The Practical Guide: Identification, Evaluation, and Treatment of Overweight and Obesity in Adults (NIH Obesity Guide) published in 2000.

My bout with ovarian cancer interrupted my plan to continue this trend. The dietician at the Cancer Center was adamant that I maintain my weight during chemotherapy. Unfortunately after I completed chemotherapy I continued to gain. I am trying get back on track.

Making **healthy food choices** is important. The Food Guide Pyramid is a good place to start. Over the years the essential features of nutritional advice has been modified. The original Basic Seven Food Groups were reduced to the Basic Four Food Groups. Later the Food Guide Pyramid replaced the Basic Four. The current Food Guide Pyramid is under criticism for two major reasons.

The first major criticism is that the current Food Guide Pyramid doesn't provide sufficient information about the relationship between the ingestion of animal fats and increased low-density lipoprotein (LDL) or "bad cholesterol." In addition, it doesn't address trans fatty acids—a newcomer to the list of foods to avoid. Until all manufacturers include the amount of trans fatty acids on food labels, reading food labels and avoiding hydrogenated fats or fats that remain solid at room temperature is prudent.

The second major criticism is that the current Food Guide Pyramid doesn't address the glycemic index of carbohydrates. Starches and sugars with high glycemic loads elevate blood glucose level rapidly and excessively and trigger the secretion of insulin to reverse high blood glucose levels. Hunger returns within a few hours and we eat more. In the meantime, current recommendations include not eating large quantities of foods that have a high glycemic index (including some cereals, white breads, white rice, and baked potatoes).

Many experts point out that 35% of cancer and cancer deaths are related to poor dietary practices. They support the recommendations of the National Cancer Institute (NCI), the American Cancer Society (ACS), and the American Institute for Cancer Research (AICR) to use foods from plant sources and fiber and to limit food from animal sources. They endorse the use of foods low in fat and salt and high in antioxidants and phytochemicals. Foods high in polyunsaturated fats produce free radicals that have the potential to disrupt cells and alter DNA producing cancer. Antioxidants neutralize free radicals and prevent this cell disruption. Eating a variety of fruits and a rainbow of vegetables provides these antioxidants. Heavy alcohol use may result in serious vitamin and mineral deficiencies and is not recommended.

According to the NIH Obesity Guide one of the complications of obesity that primary health care providers need to search for is cancer—colorectal and prostate cancer in men and endometrial, gallbladder, cervical, ovarian, and breast cancer in women. The consensus of the Expert Panel that developed the guideline is that those of us who are seriously overweight need to be self-motivated to initiate weight loss regimens under the direction of our primary health care providers.

Following the Panel's guidelines reduces a person's chances of being diagnosed with cancer. No guarantees! Early detection and treatment of cancer is crucial. Prudent people carry out periodic examinations of the skin, genital self-examination and breast self-examination. Prudent women visit their primary health care provider or gynecologist for an annual clinical vaginal exam and Pap smear, clinical breast examination and mammogram. They contact their primary health care provider or gynecologist at once if they become aware of any cancer warning sign. Signs include unusual bleeding or discharge, change in bowel or bladder habits, sores that fail to heal, indigestion or difficulty swallowing, obvious change in mole or wart, nagging cough or hoarseness, or thickening or lump in breast or elsewhere.

Prudent women will contact their primary health care provider or gynecologist immediately if they experience any ovarian cancer symptom that lasts more than 2–3 weeks. These include: bloating, a feeling of fullness, gas, frequent or urgent urination, nausea, indigestion, constipation, diarrhea, menstrual disorders, pain during intercourse, fatigue, backaches (National Ovarian Cancer Coalition: 1-888-ovarian or www.ovarian.org). Initial work-ups include a vaginal and rectal examination, a CA 125 blood test, and a transvaginal sonogram or ultrasound. Work-ups may also involve computerized tomography (CT) scanning and magnetic resonance imaging (MRI).

Most women hope that all this fuss will come to naught. Perhaps they hope that nothing will be found and that they'll be thrown off the speeding train into a soft pile of hay. Then they'll get up and brush off their clothing and head for home, family, and friends and a life interrupted.

After all, this happened to me in 1985. The lump in my breast was nothing. The physician was happy that he could give me good news. He had nothing but bad news for the other people whom he saw that day.

The situation was different for me in 2001. Instead of making the day for my primary care provider, she was being bombarded with glimpses into my upcoming journey and struggling to insure that I didn't get on the wrong train. The journey is an unwelcome but necessary one for many women. Only women who are vigilant—have health screenings and/or seek follow-up when warnings are sounded—have the opportunity to embark on a journey with a potentially successful outcome.

In the past most Americans didn't have a primary care provider who gave immunizations and did health examinations and periodic health screenings.

Instead when they were sick, they sought the assistance of the neighborhood pharmacist or physician.

My family didn't take me to see a physician unless I was ill. My mother diagnosed measles when I was five. She isolated me from my playmates and carefully protected my eyes from the sunlight. When I was eight my eardrums burst and the neighborhood physician came to the house. He couldn't do much because penicillin wasn't available yet.

I had a rash when I was 13. My mother relied on the Collier's Family Medical Guide and decided that it was German measles. She kept me home from school for the recommended isolation period. This unnerved the school nurse because she didn't have physician clearance for me to return to school. Years later I learned that I had a rubella antibody titer that confirmed immunity. My mother's diagnosis had been on target.

During my nursing school years I obtained most of my health care from the school physician and I saw my own physician sporadically for episodic care until he died. After college I moved about and saw local physicians for episodic care. In the late 1970s I became concerned that my overall medical care was disjointed. I set out to establish myself with a physician who would see me on a regular basis. A nurse whom I met at a critical care conference recommended a few excellent physicians. I chose the internist who also concentrated on endocrinology because several people in my family had diabetes. He did my first gynecologic examinations. My health insurance didn't include well adult care. After he enlisted in the army I needed to find another physician.

I located another internist in the area. His focus was the heart. At this time my health insurance covered well adult care but it didn't cover routine gynecologic examinations by a gynecologist. This physician provided vaginal examinations and Pap smears on a regular basis and always assured me that things looked good. When health insurance coverage became available for gynecologic examinations with a gynecologist, I didn't consider changing my past practice. This physician wasn't aware that I was at high risk for ovarian cancer. Later he left his practice to specialize in in-hospital cardiology.

When I had my first gynecologic examination with my current primary care provider, she was very thorough but she didn't express concern. However, she didn't know my baseline because her staff didn't obtain my medical record. She couldn't have known that the mass in my pelvic region that was making me uncomfortable was growing and not regressing. She wouldn't have the opportunity to realize this on my next examination because I had a symptom that demanded my attention.

Mary her receptionist knew that I needed to be seen. Although the nurse practitioner didn't know that the mass was cancer, she saw to it that appropriate tests were ordered. When the test results started to come in, my current primary care provider had to run to catch up with the speeding train. For me recognizing and reacting to the symptom was crucial.

Most women who develop ovarian cancer don't have the symptom that I had—I had unexpected bleeding. Instead they have unclear symptoms that are likely to be ignored. The National Ovarian Cancer Coalition describes the onset of ovarian cancer as a whispering. Women must learn to listen for its whispers.

Women, who are at high risk and have their health care orchestrated by a general practitioner or internist, need to have gynecologic examinations with a gynecologist. Women whose menstrual cycles haven't been interrupted for pregnancy are at high risk. Gynecologists are more in tune to the subtle symptoms of ovarian cancer. Older women and immigrant women who've only seen a physician when they are ill need to know why seeing a physician when they aren't ill is also vital to their well-being.

In November 2003 I attended a conference on Women's Health. Another woman at the conference told me, My mother would never have a GYN exam. She died of an undiagnosed lower abdominal problem that I suspect could've been a GYN cancer." As the conversation progressed, she went on to say, "My own GYN exam is long overdue. I'm trying to get up the courage to have one."

I told her that I could understand how she felt. I thought that I no longer needed to have gynecologic examinations. I had three consecutive negative pap tests and wasn't sexually active. My primary physician had insisted on doing a complete examination. Although I didn't have cervical or vaginal cancer, having a record of a recent examination had expedited my follow-up when I had my first symptom. My ovarian cancer had been detected before it spread to surrounding tissue. I encouraged her to avoid procrastinating any longer.

15

Heart-rending Memorabilia of an Uninvited Journey

No one wants to take the uninvited journey into the world of being a person who has cancer. One in every two men and one in every three women do. The uninvited journey is different in many ways for all of us yet similar in other ways. The journey with cancer infringes on our lives and attempts to derail us from our life's major pathways. Those who have gone with us and will continue to go with us on our unique life journeys influence our responses to this unwelcome intrusion into our lives. What does it matter that we don't know where the journey will take or what will happen on the journey? They come with us.

The current approaches to treatment of cancers are varied and complex. Research protocols are being continuously developed and studied. Approaches to the treatment of cancer are constantly being modified. When women learn that they may have cancer, they need to make decisions about treatment. They need to make decisions at a time when they are thunderstruck from the news of the potential diagnosis.

Traditional modes of cancer treatment have included surgery, chemotherapy, and radiation therapy. Newer modes include biological therapy and radioimmune therapy. Although I didn't know which cancer I had until after surgery, I discovered a helpful resource—*Everyone's Guide to Cancer Therapy: How Cancer Is Diagnosed, Treated, and Managed Day to Day* by Dollinger, Rosenbaum, and Cable. Inasmuch as I had no reproductive function to preserve, I had no qualms about surgery. I told my gynecologic oncologist to take it all out. I don't regret that decision.

About six months after my surgery and diagnosis a colleague called me to see how I was doing. She told me that she'd been diagnosed with ovarian cancer during her reproductive years. She was able to delay her treatment until after she gave birth to her daughter. She told me that it was "very difficult, unbelievable, just awful". Women who discover that they have ovarian cancer during their child-bearing years need to discuss their potential choices with their gynecologic oncologist.

Unintended or toxic effects that may necessitate changes in the protocols and symptom management accompany cancer treatment protocols. Agents that search for and destroy cancer cells also affect normal cells. The National Cancer Institute (NCI) has developed clinical toxicity criteria (CTC) that guide clinicians as they as they adjust dose and frequency of chemotherapy or radiation therapy. Clinicians may prescribe an array of cytoprotectants (cell protectors) or medications that may limit or prevent these effects. The purpose of cell protectors is to defend cells or tissue against undesired effects and to enable the continuation of prescribed doses at prescribed intervals. Research that attempts to determine the effectiveness of cell protectors is ongoing. Some cell protectors are pharmaceuticals. Others are found in natural sources. I learned that glutathione that is found in raw vegetables such as carrots and broccoli is also available as a medication. The medication is being studied in clinical trials for its effectiveness in modulating cisplatin-induced neurotoxicity. Thus far, the Food and Drug Administration (FDA) has not approved glutathione for this use.

Although I was in the first stage (the cancer was confined to the ovaries and hadn't spread), it was a grade III cell—a very aggressive tumor. My oncologists prescribed a standard course of treatment—carboplatin (Paraplatin) and paclitaxel (Taxol) every three weeks for six cycles. Their intent was that I receive the prescribed doses of these drugs at the prescribed intervals. They intended to monitor me closely because a variety of unintended effects accompany the use of these and other drugs that comprise the anti-cancer war chest.

Ricky explained that diverse unintended effects might plague me during my chemotherapy. She also shared numerous tricks of the trade that the staff at the Cancer Center uses to minimize them. She also told me about serious effects that could interfere with my receiving the prescribed doses of chemotherapy drugs at the prescribed intervals.

In addition, while I was traveling on the high-speed express train, I discovered many interesting tidbits in the journals that arrive at my home each month. One of these was an article about ovarian cancer for nurses. If I answered the accompanying test, I could earn continuing education credits to meet state nursing license requirements. I completed the test and received a certificate. An influx of educational materials and journals that expanded my knowledge about cancer research also began to arrive in my home.

Some research reports describe efforts to prevent or manage the unintended effects of chemotherapy drugs. For example, during chemotherapy and/or other treatment methods the bone marrow that produces various blood cells stops producing these cells. Insufficient production of red blood cells, white blood cells, and platelets may result in fatigue related to anemia, infection, and bleeding.

Until recently transfusions were needed to treat severe anemia. The development of recombinant DNA human erythropoetin (epoetin alfa) given one-three times a week to stimulate red blood cell production has lessened the need for transfusion. Currently, darbepoetin alfa—a product that may be given every two weeks—is being used to reverse anemia. Ongoing clinical trials to determine if darbepoetin alfa will prevent the decrease in red blood cells are taking place.

Epoetin alfa and darbepoetin alfa are only useful for anemia triggered by cancer treatment. Transfusions are still necessary in cancer-related anemia because the fewer red blood cells that are produced have a shorter lifespan.

In addition decreased white blood cells during cancer treatment may result in increased susceptibility to infection. Filgrastin (Neupogen) may be used to stimulate immature white blood cells to divide and mature. Recently, pegfilgrastin—a product that is effective when given less frequently—has become available. Clinical trials to determine if the decrease in white blood cells can be prevented are ongoing.

Decreased platelet production may also accompany chemotherapy and may result in increased bleeding. Oprelvekin (Neumega), a new product that stimulates platelet production has only recently been available.

Nausea and vomiting are troubling unwelcome intrusions in the life of persons undergoing chemotherapy. Recent articles in the Journal of Supportive

Oncology have described the various facets of the problem and recent progress in its management. As oncologists refine their scientific knowledge of the physiology of nausea and vomiting and study the effects of newly developed medications, they're able to provide a more systematic approach to management of chemotherapy-induced nausea and vomiting (CINV).

Chemotherapy drugs vary in their emetic potential (the possibility that they'll trigger nausea and vomiting). In the absence of preventive antiemetic treatment, Carboplatin has moderate emetic potential and Paclitaxel has low emetic potential. Several oncology groups have developed guidelines for antiemetic treatment.

Multiple nerve pathways are involved in chemotherapy-induced nausea and vomiting (CINV). Several classes of drugs that interfere with transmission of nerve impulses have been developed and have improved the available supportive care to patients undergoing cancer treatment.

Medications known as serotonin-3 antagonists ($5HT_3$) are recommended in combination with a corticosteroid to prevent the acute CINV that occurs within the first 24 hours. One of these medications had been prescribed for me. I received this drug intravenously prior to chemotherapy and took it orally twice daily for seven doses. I followed the instructions precisely. It was effective.

Apparently controlling acute CINV also controls the delayed CINV that occurs after 24 hours and lasts longer. It also controls the anticipatory CINV that occurs before next course of chemotherapy. Medications classified as dopamine antagonists may be prescribed for delayed or breakthrough CINV. Although prochlorperazine was prescribed for me, I didn't need to use it.

Those who have breakthrough symptoms need to take the prescribed drug immediately and not delay in the hopes that the symptoms will go away. The symptoms have no place to go! If the drugs that have been prescribed are ineffective, promptly notifying the designated health care provider is crucial. Preventing the loss of essential salts and fluids is crucial to recovery from cancer.

Having chemotherapy-induced nausea and vomiting may precipitate anticipatory nausea or vomiting prior to future chemotherapy. Women who had cancer treatment before the newer drugs that control nausea and vomiting became available have described their dreaded experiences with anticipatory nausea and vomiting.

Unfortunately some people may have refractory CINV—when preventive and rescue drugs fail in early cycles, symptoms persist during later cycles. Others may have nausea and vomiting that is related to their cancer rather than its treatment. My hospital roommate had nausea and vomited repeatedly. She didn't tell me whether her symptoms were related to the chemotherapy or to her cancer.

Overall remarkable progress has been made. Research to identify other neurotransmitters that may be involved in CINV and discover other potentially effective medications is ongoing. Sources: Navari (Journal of Supportive Oncology, July-August 2003) and Grunberg, SM (Journal of Supportive Oncology, January-February 2004, Supplement)

Unrelieved pain is a potentially devastating experience for people who have cancer. Patients and their caretakers need to know that pain relief is available.

Pain may be related to the primary tumors or to secondary metastases. Surgery, chemotherapy, or radiation therapy may induce pain. Often cancer-related pain is produced by invasion of bone or soft tissue resulting in compression of blood vessels or nerves. Numerous analgesics (pain relievers) have been developed. Acceptable pain relief is available. Those who have pain need to pursue pain relief actively. When they find it, they need to view it as a treasure that they will not let go.

Pain status is now taken into account as the fifth vital sign. Failure of health care providers to assess pain and provide adequate pain relief is unacceptable! An appropriate pain scale based on the individual's age and cognitive level is used. Recently I received a bookmark copy of the FACES scale in the mail. My niece thought that a person in pain was supposed to make a face that resembled the face on the FACES scale. She asked me if her facial expression matched the face on the scale. I explained that children would point to the face that would reveal how much their pain hurt. Most commonly a person is asked to rate his or her pain on a scale of 0–10 where "0" is "no pain" and "10" is the "worst pain imaginable".

People who are in pain may be apathetic, crying, irritable, or grimacing. They may be inactive, or fail to move extremities or wince with movement. People who have acute or chronic pain may not always exhibit symptoms of arousal—changes in alertness or in vital signs.

A variety of non-narcotic pain relievers, narcotic pain relievers, and drugs that enhance the effects of pain relievers are available. The unique pain management approach depends on patient's current status and the type of pain—acute or chronic. A pain management consulting team may be involved in designing the pain management approach for some patients.

Patient controlled analgesia (PCA) is commonly used to allay acute pain after surgery as this approach adapts to individual variation in responses. A microprocessor infusion pump is used to deliver precise doses to the person who is experiencing pain. After an initial higher dose, a lower maintenance dose is prescribed. The patient is able to activate the prescribed dosing within the preset lockout interval.

If severe acute pain is present, repeated intravenous boluses (concentrated doses) may be used to provide relief, followed by a maintenance infusion. Continuous intravenous infusion may be used in chronic pain management. Provision of additional boluses (intermittent larger doses) to manage breakthrough pain should be available. Increasing the rate of infusion may be needed. Whenever possible, an oral drug is preferred for the treatment of chronic pain.

Non-narcotic pain relievers may be used for the management of mild or moderate pain. If pain is severe, the use of a slow release narcotic is needed. Initially a rapid release narcotic is given for 48 hours to learn the average daily dosing requirement. Then a slow release narcotic for two-thirds of the estimated daily dose may be prescribed. Extra rapid release narcotic doses would be nearby and could be taken anytime.

An analgesic adjuvant (aid to the pain reliever) may be used to manage a specific side effect of a narcotic drug. For example, a scopolamine skin patch may be prescribed to reduce nausea and vomiting or caffeine may be prescribed during the day to reverse daytime sleepiness.

The constipation effect of the narcotic pain reliever compels the use of a bowel regimen—usually, a stool softener, such as docusate, and a laxative, such as senna. Continuing the bowel regimen while the patient is receiving a continuous narcotic pain relief is crucial. In the future drugs that interfere with the effect of narcotics on the bowel may be available.

Currently people who use narcotic pain relievers inevitably have constipation and need to maintain a continuous bowel regimen. Failure to do so may result in intestinal obstruction and hospitalization. Frequently narcotic pain relievers are discontinued during hospitalization and may not be put back in place upon discharge. As a result patients suffer. Continuing the bowel regimen while narcotic pain relievers are being used is crucial. Preventing serious intestinal slowdown and hospitalization is the way to go!

Constipation is also a common side effect of some chemotherapy agents. Constipation may be managed by walking, by drinking 8–10 cups of liquid daily, and by eating a high-fiber diet and snacks. Using stool softeners and laxatives as directed by the oncology center may be necessary. If constipation is severe or persists, contact the designated health care provider.

Diarrhea is also a common side effect of some chemotherapy agents. Diarrhea may be managed by drinking sufficient fluid to replace losses between meals, by eating foods that are high in potassium to replace losses, and by limiting whole grain cereals and breads, fruits and vegetables with seeds and skin.

Broth, gelatin, apple or cranberry juice, diluted orange juice, bananas, applesauce, dry white toast or crackers, boiled white rice, or potato may be helpful. If diarrhea persists, contact the designated health care provider. I was told to call if diarrhea persisted more than 2–3 days.

In 2003 Saltz pointed out in Supportive Oncology (May/Jun) that the National Cancer Institute has developed and updated criteria that define diarrhea based on an increase in the number of bowel movements over baseline. He emphasizes the importance of determining difference between the patient's normal pattern and the changes in the form and frequency of movements. Early detection of impending dehydration and administration of fluids in an outpatient setting may prevent inpatient admission and the need for more aggressive management.

Mucositis or inflammation of the lining of the mouth and throat may occur during chemotherapy or radiation to the head or neck. Brushing teeth with a soft toothbrush, using non-alcoholic mouthwash, and using a water-pik may prevent injury. If inflammation occurs, using a baking soda and water paste and/or rinsing with warm salt water have been suggested. Eating warm or cool soft foods and avoiding salty, coarse or spicy foods and citrus is recommended. Drinking liquids with food is helpful. If mouth pain is severe or progressive, contact the designated health care provider. Local anesthetic agents that may be used on a short time basis may be recommended.

Fatigue may result from anemia or from emotional distress, pain, sleep disturbance, the disease itself, or its treatment (Mock in Given, 2003). In comparison to healthy individuals, the fatigue experience associated with cancer is more intense and not apt to be relieved by usual measures. Fatigue has been described as having many dimensions and may include weakness, lack of concentration, and lack of motivation. While Rosenbaum says that fatigue is disproportionate to effort, Mock reports an inverse correlation between fatigue level and activity level. Unrelieved fatigue interferes with daily activities and compromises quality of life.

The approach to fatigue is guided by its source. Mock points out the importance of assessing the factors that contribute to fatigue. These include pain, emotional distress, anemia, sleep disturbance, and thyroid function. She goes on to say that other contributors in cancer patients—water and salt imbalances, heart and breathing ailments, and undernourishment—also need to be addressed.

Mock reviewed a number of research studies, including her own, that examined the effort of exercise on fatigue. Exercise interventions included the use of stationary bicycles, home-based walking and low intensity aerobics. She reported that those who exercised had significantly lower levels of fatigue than those who didn't.

Arthralgia and myalgia (joint and muscle pain) may accompany chemotherapy with paclitaxel. The information that I was given was that it might occur within a few days of being treated and disappear within a week. In 1998 Savarese and colleagues found that five patients who reported joint and muscle aches after their first round of paclitaxel took glutamine after their second round and didn't report joint and muscle aches after their next round. Ricky suggested that I use glutamine three times a day for four days. She said that glutamine could be purchased in the local health food store.

Glutamine is available as a caplet and in powder form. Initially I bought caplets. I had to take 10 caplets three times a day. I had difficulty drinking the amount of water that I needed to swallow 10 caplets. My niece helped me to split the caplets into smaller portions so I could swallow them with less water. Later I purchased the powder. I was surprised to learn that I'd be using two heaping tablespoons of the powder. As a nurse I was used to precise measurement. However, the powder dissolved easily in orange juice. Although the color wasn't appealing, the mixture was palatable.

In my case approximately 48 hours after receiving paclitaxel I couldn't rest my feet on a soft sofa. The only measure that provided relief from discomfort was using a pillow under my legs to prevent my feet from touching the surface.

In 2003 Jacobson and colleagues (Journal of Supportive Oncology, Nov/Dec) report using a crossover design to randomly assigned 36 patients who'd previously reported arthralgia or myalgia after paclitaxel to receive either glutamine or placebo on their next round. On the following round all participants received the alternate substance. Jacob and colleagues didn't find evidence that using glutamine was beneficial. These findings didn't surprise me, but the sample was small. I would like to see the results of other studies.

Peripheral neuropathy (tingling, burning, or numbness of the feet, hands, or mouth) may accompany chemotherapy with carboplatin. Although Paice discussed other common neuropathic pain syndromes in 2003 (Supportive Oncology, Jul/Aug), I only mention chemotherapy-induced neuropathy related to platin drugs here.

The information that I was given was that symptoms might increase with each cycle but they usually resolve after treatment is over. Ricky suggested that I use vitamin B6 50 mg three times a day. Vitamin B6 tablets are available in most local pharmacies but the vitamin is absorbed quickly and eliminated quickly. I decided to use a higher dose slow release caplet and hoped that it would provide lasting relief. I took it twice a day. Although I didn't experience total relief, the vitamin seemed to help. When I decided to reduce the dose, my symptoms got worse. I continued to take vitamin B6 for a long time before I started to reduce the dose gradually.

In the meantime I read somewhere that platinum is deposited in the dorsal ganglia (clusters of cell bodies of sensory nerves located along the posterior roots of spinal nerves) and thus causes neuropathy. I knew that the chickenpox and other related viruses remained dormant in the dorsal ganglia and flared up during periods of heat and stress. During my search for a solution to my persistent peripheral neuropathy, I learned that glutathione may be helpful but it works best if taken in natural sources rather than in supplements. Some of the best sources are uncooked broccoli and carrots. The amount that is suggested can be obtained by eating 1–2 raw medium carrots or 8–10 raw mini-carrots daily. This seems to help me and I am still eating raw carrots.

If I lie on my back at night, the weight of covers still hurts my toes. Sometimes I have carpal pedal spasms in my 2nd and 3rd toes. If I work too long at the computer or at other fine work, my fingers get a little tingly. Fortunately, my symptoms are gradually diminishing.

Blocked tear ducts were an unexpected finding. Neither the various drug handbooks nor Ricky mentioned this possibility. Nonetheless an article by Saaditi in 2003 (The American Journal of Oncology Review, Nov/Dec) reported that secretion of docetaxel into tears may contribute to blockage of the tear ducts. Apparently the problem is related to the frequency of dosing of the chemotherapy agent.

Often while I was working in the garden in late May or early June 2002, my eyes would fill up with dense tears. The experience resembled looking at the world through an oily substance. I was compelled to go inside frequently and wash my hands so that I could flush my eyes. For convenience I purchased Refresh Plus an over the counter preservative free lubricant eye solution that provided relief. The lubricant came in individual vials and I could take a vial with me. I could feel a gritty substance whenever I massaged my tear ducts.

If I'd suspected that this could be related to chemotherapy, I would've reported it to my oncologists. The problem resolved spontaneously by July 31st and I didn't mention it to my ophthalmologist.

A series of nosebleeds diverted my attention. The first and only consequential episode took place on July 12th. On a scale of one to ten, it was definitely a ten! The remaining episodes that occurred 1–3 times a week until August 19th could be rated as two, three, or five. The "basis" of the nosebleeds was unclear but "may" have been related to changes in the mucosa during chemotherapy. Platelet counts weren't low enough to account for this intrusion.

My ophthalmologist did note that I had mild cataracts but he hadn't told me this at the time. When I returned for my annual eye examination one year later, the receptionist asked for a referral from my primary care provider because I had cataracts. He told me that I did have mild cataracts but they hadn't progressed. I haven't read that the chemotherapy medications that were prescribed for me would cause cataracts.

For the most part I weathered the unwanted journey without too much difficulty but others who were going on this unwanted journey weren't fairing as well.

16

Passing the Torch

Things are definitely settling down. The train is pulling very, very slowly into the station. I think that I'm going to be able to disembark. If this were any other disease, I wouldn't even have a second thought. But this is cancer. Not all cancer is curable. Apparently some cancers are curable.

My oncologists have been optimistic because I've been in the best prognosis group. I expect to do well but nonetheless I'll maintain a heightened vigilance. The SMART Study ended in February 2004. The data is being analyzed and the medical community will learn of its outcomes.

The Women's Health Study that I have participated in since 1993 ended in March 2004. I learned that I have been taking Vitamin E and not a placebo and low dose aspirin and not a placebo. I anticipate learning about the results of this study as well.

In February 2004 the Ovarian Cancer Education Awareness Network (OCEAN) celebrated its fourth anniversary. After they presented a check for $500,000.00 to MGH for ovarian cancer research, Arlan Fuller and Michael Seiden spoke briefly about accomplishments that have been supported by the efforts of OCEAN.

Dr. Fuller discussed the need to expand on the knowledge discovered during the Human Genome Project. He explained the limitations of current microscopic techniques used in pathology for predicting who will survive, who won't survive, and who'll have successful outcomes after relapse with current standard treatment. He emphasized the importance of differentiating genetic sequences that identify those who do well and those who don't do well with various protocols. This knowledge will enable clinicians to tailor their approaches to their individual patients.

Dr Seiden highlighted the research being done by David Livingston at Dana Farber to identify these important gene sequences. He emphasized that the important contribution of the tumor bank initiated by OCEAN in supporting his research.

Dr. Seiden also mentioned the promise of improved screening tests or potential early markers of ovarian cancer as works in progress. He cited one of these early markers as being potentially more useful than the CA 125 antigen. If the ongoing research confirms its usefulness, this knowledge will enable clinicians to detect ovarian cancer in earlier stages.

To be designated as more useful than the CA 125 as an early marker or indicator of ovarian cancer a screening test would have to meet specific criteria. The screening test would need to have better sensitivity (identify ovarian cancer when it is present) and better specificity (rule out ovarian cancer when it is not present) than the CA 125 has. The ideal screening test or early marker would have optimal sensitivity and specificity and would differentiate between women who need a diagnostic work-up and those who do not.

Typically screening tests don't have 100% sensitivity and 100% specificity. The objective of ongoing research is find an indicator that won't send too many women who are disease-free for further work-up while it doesn't fail to send those who have disease for essential follow-up.

The CA 125 antigen has low sensitivity and low specificity. This test may fail to identify too many women who have ovarian cancer and may not rule out too many women who don't have ovarian cancer.

In 1968 when Rita (a champion survivor) had ovarian cancer, nitrogen mustard and radiation comprised her treatment. According to Arlan Fuller only one drug was available to treat ovarian cancer in the 1960s and now thirty drugs are available (in Synergy Winter 2004). In 1968 when Rita had third stage ovarian cancer, survival was unusual and now more women are surviving. As scientists unravel the genetic sequences underlying ovarian cancer and develop earlier indicators of ovarian cancer, early detection and more targeted treatment will be possible. Survival rates will improve.

In June 2004 I walked for the North Shore Cancer Center for the first time. The names of my surviving and non-surviving friends and acquaintances and my supporters accompanied me. I was amazed by the numbers of people who turned out for this event. I hope to be able to continue to take part in this activity.

As I reflect on how I chose to tell the story of my journey, I realize that entering into the experience of being on the other side of the looking glass didn't come easy. During my struggles to make sense of the strangely familiar surroundings, I could interpret events from a nurse's perspective and translate complex information into simple explanations that I could share with other women and their significant others. My struggles enabled me to gain a greater understanding of their experiences. I am grateful to those who've told me that they or their loved ones have made it though their ordeal. They shared their hope with me. Now I share my hope with others. My shared story ends but my journey continues.

Sources and Resources

INTERNET

American Cancer Society
800-ACS-2345
www.cancer.org

American Institute for Cancer Research
800-841-8114
www.aicr.org

National Cancer Institute
800-4cancer
www.cancer.gov

NCI Glossary
www.cancer.gov/dictionary/

National Ovarian Cancer Coalition
888-OVARIAN
www.ovarian.org

American Pain Foundation
www.painfoundation.org
1-888-615-PAIN

American Pain Society
www.ampainsoc.org
1-847-375-4715

National Pain Foundation
www.painconnection.org

LITERATURE

Songs from a Lead-lined Room: Notes—High and Low—From my Journey through Breast Cancer and Radiation, by Suzanne Strempek Shea (Beacon Press, 2002).

No Time to Die: Living with Ovarian Cancer, by Liz Tilberis (Avon books, 1998).

Evidence-Based Cancer Care and Prevention: Behavioral Interventions, Edited by C. W. Given and associates, 2003.

Cancer Support: Total Quality Management in 2003. Jointly sponsored by the Dannemiller Memorial Educational Foundation and the McMahon Publishing Center.

References to journal articles have not been included for a few reasons. The primary one is that research is ongoing and more recent research reports will likely be available. In addition, the primary intent of the author for including "souvenirs" is to describe her discoveries during the journey rather than to present a summary of the available research. It is difficult to do justice to the array of cancer research, as cancer research is an expansive and rapidly changing dynamic field of inquiry.

Acknowledgments

To the many caring, compassionate, and competent people who provided for me on my journey:

Linda Rosenbaum Duska M. D., the staff of the Gillette Center, the Surgical Center, Bigelow Seven, and Nuclear Medicine at the Massachusetts General Hospital in Boston,

Joel Schwartz M. D., and the staff at the North Shore Cancer Center in Peabody, Massachusetts,

To Suzanne Strempek Shea who impressed me with the importance of sharing this story

To Mary Burke D. N. Sc. who not only listened to my story but also poured over the manuscript and made suggestions

To the Harvard Medical Faculty who created and offered an elective course titled Living with a Life Threatening Illness for first year medical students and to the medical student who listened ardently to my story

To those who joined me on my journey, I express my sincere gratitude

Some names in this book have been changed to protect privacy.
Alex
Amanda
Barry
Bud
Dee
Faith
Jayne
Jim
Josh
Kyle
Marie
Pam
Paula
Tim
Tom
Robin
Sally
Sharon G
Zachary

Other names in the book are actual names.

978-0-595-34709-4
0-595-34709-6